DISABILITY STUDIES

NEURAL PLASTICITY IN CHRONIC PAIN

DISABILITY STUDIES

JOAV MERRICK - SERIES EDITOR –
NATIONAL INSTITUTE OF CHILD HEALTH
AND HUMAN DEVELOPMENT,
MINISTRY OF SOCIAL AFFAIRS, JERUSALEM

Contemporary Issues in Intellectual Disabilities
V.P. Prasher (Editor)
2010. ISBN: 978-1-61668-023-7 (Hardcover)
2010. ISBN: 978-1-61209-292-8 (E-book)

**Disability from a Humanistic Perspective: Towards a Better
Quality of Life**
Shunit Reiter
2011. ISBN: 978-1-60456-412-9

Pain Management Yearbook 2009
Joav Merrick (Editor)
2011. ISBN: 978-1-61209-666-7

Pain. Brain Stimulation in the Treatment of Pain
Helena Knotkova, Ricardo Cruciani and Joav Merrick (Editors)
2011. ISBN: 978-1-60876-690-1 (Hardcover)
2011. ISBN: 978-1-61470-495-9 (E-book)

**Cancer in Children and Adults with Intellectual Disabilities:
Current Research Aspects**
Daniel Satgé and Joav Merrick (Editors)
2011. ISBN: 978-1-61761-856-7 (Hardcover)
2011. ISBN: 978-1-61122-187-9 (E-book)

Rett Syndrome: Therapeutic Interventions
Meir Lotan and Joav Merrick (Editors)
2011. ISBN: 978-1-61728-614-8 (Hardcover)
2011. ISBN: 978-1-61761-131-5 (E-book)

Pain Management Yearbook 2010
Joav Merrick (Editor)
2011. ISBN: 978-1-61209-972-9

Neural Plasticity in Chronic Pain
Helena Knotkova, Ricardo A. Cruciani and Joav Merrick (Editors)
2012. ISBN: 978-1-61324-657-3

DISABILITY STUDIES

NEURAL PLASTICITY IN CHRONIC PAIN

HELENA KNOTKOVA
RICARDO A. CRUCIANI
AND
JOAV MERRICK
EDITORS

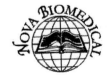

Nova Science Publishers, Inc.
New York

Copyright © 2012 by Nova Science Publishers, Inc.

All rights reserved. No part of this book may be reproduced, stored in a retrieval system or transmitted in any form or by any means: electronic, electrostatic, magnetic, tape, mechanical photocopying, recording or otherwise without the written permission of the Publisher.

For permission to use material from this book please contact us:
Telephone 631-231-7269; Fax 631-231-8175
Web Site: http://www.novapublishers.com

NOTICE TO THE READER

The Publisher has taken reasonable care in the preparation of this book, but makes no expressed or implied warranty of any kind and assumes no responsibility for any errors or omissions. No liability is assumed for incidental or consequential damages in connection with or arising out of information contained in this book. The Publisher shall not be liable for any special, consequential, or exemplary damages resulting, in whole or in part, from the readers' use of, or reliance upon, this material. Any parts of this book based on government reports are so indicated and copyright is claimed for those parts to the extent applicable to compilations of such works.

Independent verification should be sought for any data, advice or recommendations contained in this book. In addition, no responsibility is assumed by the publisher for any injury and/or damage to persons or property arising from any methods, products, instructions, ideas or otherwise contained in this publication.

This publication is designed to provide accurate and authoritative information with regard to the subject matter covered herein. It is sold with the clear understanding that the Publisher is not engaged in rendering legal or any other professional services. If legal or any other expert assistance is required, the services of a competent person should be sought. FROM A DECLARATION OF PARTICIPANTS JOINTLY ADOPTED BY A COMMITTEE OF THE AMERICAN BAR ASSOCIATION AND A COMMITTEE OF PUBLISHERS.

Additional color graphics may be available in the e-book version of this book.

Library of Congress Cataloging-in-Publication Data

Neural plasticity in chronic pain / editors, Helena Knotkova, Ricardo A. Cruciani, Joav Merrick.
     p. ; cm. -- (Disability studies series)
  Includes bibliographical references and index.
  ISBN 978-1-61324-657-3 (hardcover)
  1. Chronic pain--Pathophysiology. 2. Neuroplasticity. I. Knotkova, Helena. II. Cruciani, Ricardo. III. Merrick, Joav, 1950- IV. Series: Disability studies (Nova Science Publishers)
  [DNLM: 1. Pain--physiopathology. 2. Chronic Disease. 3. Neuronal Plasticity--physiology. WL 704]
  RB127.N45 2011
  616'.0472--dc23

2011015624

Published by Nova Science Publishers, Inc. ✛ New York

Contents

Preface		**ix**
Foreword	*Russell K. Portenoy*	**xi**
Introduction:	Neural plasticity in chronic pain *Helena Knotkova, Ricardo A Cruciani, and Joav Merrick*	**xv**
Chapter I	Targeting TRPV1 for pain relief *Marcello Trevisani, and Arpad Szallasi*	**1**
Chapter II	Allodynia and neuronal plasticity *Ricardo A Cruciani, Charles B Stacy, Seth Resnik and Helena Knotkova*	**33**
Chapter III	Spinal cord neural plasticity in chronic pain and its clinical implication *Jacqueline R Dauch, and Hsinlin T Cheng*	**47**
Chapter IV	The role of neuroimaging in chronic pain syndromes *Christine Chang, and Marco Pappagallo*	**69**
Chapter V	Sensorimotor training and its implication for cortical reorganization *Martin Diers, and Herta Flor*	**77**
Chapter VI	The role of mental imagery in chronic deafferentation pain and its effect on cortical reorganization *Kate MacIver, Paul Sacco, and Turo Nurmikko*	**91**

Chapter VII	Functional and structural cortical neuroplasticity in trigeminal neuropathic pain *Marcos FH DosSantos, and Alexandre F DaSilva*	**107**
Chapter VIII	Brain stimulation for the treatment of neuropathic facial pain *Helena Knotkova, Arash Nafissi, Eliah Soto, Dirk Rasche, and Ricardo A Cruciani*	**131**
Chapter IX	Neuroplasticity in carpal tunnel syndrome *Vitaly Napadow, Yumi Maeda, Joseph Audette, and Norman Kettner*	**153**

Acknowledgments

Chapter X	About the editors	**185**
Chapter XI	About the Institute for Noninvasive Brain Stimulation of New York	**187**
Chapter XII	About the National Institute of Child Health and Human Development in Israel	**189**
Chapter XIII	About the disability studies book series	**193**
Index		**195**

Preface

Until recently, it was thought that the adult brain is modifiable only during early stages of ontogenesis. However, neurophysiological and neuroimaging studies now indicate that the mature human brain is under certain conditions capable of substantial neuroplastic changes. The concept of plasticity is complex and can be applied to all levels of neural organization from molecular to systemic level of neural networks. Neuroplasticity reflects the ability of human brain to alter the pattern of neural activation in response to previous experience, and recent findings indicate that the effects of experience can lead to both structural as well as functional reorganization. This book presents current research in the study of neural plasticity in chronic pain.

Foreword

*Russell K Portenoy MD**

Chairman and Gerald J. Friedman Chair in Pain Medicine and Palliative
Care, Department of Pain Medicine and Palliative Care
Beth Israel Medical Center, New York, New York, US
Professor of Neurology and Anesthesiology,
Albert Einstein College of Medicine
Chief Medical Officer, MJHS Hospice and Palliative Care

Given the mercurial maneuverings of human thought and emotion, it should
not be surprising that the central nervous system undergoes so-called "plastic"
changes in response to afferent input from a variety of internal or external
sources. Yet, until the rush of science during the past fifty years, the
extraordinary malleability of central neurons was not appreciated. The breadth
of neurobiological research during this time revealed an extraordinary capacity
for sustained changes in neuronal functioning, as well as a profound
complexity in both normal physiology and changes associated with pathology
of different types. Indeed, it seems best now to accept "neuroplasticity" as a
generic construct, or simply a descriptive that may be applied to an
exceedingly complicated group of processes that are heterogeneous at multiple
levels of analysis.

For pain researchers, this concept of neuroplasticity seems oddly parallel
to "nociception." The International Association for the Study of Pain suggests
that nociception is best defined as the "neural processes of encoding and

---

* E-mail: Rportenoy@chpnet.org

processing noxious stimuli." This definition firmly distinguishes the neural activities associated with the perception of pain from the perception itself. By using the plural of "process," and by the knowing use of both "encoding" and "processing," it indicates that the neural underpinnings of clinical pain are numerous, interacting, and involve multiple systems that subserve transmission, modulation, inhibition, or activation of other pathways. Despite its brevity, the definition says much, and it invites examination at levels that vary from the molecular to the whole person.

Such is the case with the concept of neuroplasticity. This term refers generically to a very large number of phenomena, which demand investigation at levels that extend across virtually every domain of neuroscience. It will undoubtedly require decades more to deconstruct these phenomena and apply the results to new research or to clinical medicine. Little is yet known of the variation in clinical presentation linked to stimulus-induced, prolonged changes in neuronal functioning. The effects of different types of stimuli are not apparent, and there is no appreciation for the relationship between sustained neural changes and the interactions between external and internal processes. If some of the variation in neuroplasticity relates to internal modulatory activity linked to emotions, cognitions, or concurrent events, the complexity of these processes in humans can only be imagined. Even simpler questions—what is the relationship between the imaging of neuronal activation and clinical presentation?—will require far more work. Fortunately, medicine often discovers and disseminates treatments before their modes of action are understood, and the potential for therapeutic stimulation of the nervous system will certainly forge ahead irrespective of the pace of basic science.

This volume explores some of these issues with respect to the neuroplasticity associated with noxious events, with clinical pain syndromes, and with potential pain-relieving therapies. It describes some of the fascinating changes in neuronal function observed in neuroimaging studies, and raises interesting questions about the role of neuroplastic changes in the transition from acute to chronic pain, the experience of specific symptoms such as allodynia and hyperpathia, and the potential for analgesia from cortical modulation. It describes the large variation that characterizes these changes, and in so doing, provides some insight into the enormous clinical variability in pain experience that follow similar injuries or diseases.

Each of the chapters in this volume informs both the understanding of pain specifically and broader constructs of neuroplasticity and nociception. Overall, it represents a continuing effort to relate scientific observation to human experience, and sustain the valuable dialogue between basic science and clinical medicine.

Introduction:
Neural plasticity in chronic pain

Helena Knotkova, PhD[*1,2], *Ricardo A Cruciani, MD,*
PhD[1,2,3] *and Joav Merrick, MD, MMedSci, DMSc*[4,5]

[1]Department of Pain Medicine and Palliative Care, Research Division,
Institute for Non-invasive Brain Stimulation,
Beth Israel Medical Center, New York, US
[2]Department of Neurology, Albert Einstein College of Medicine,
Bronx, New York, US
[3]Department of Anesthesiology, Albert Einstein College of Medicine,
Bronx, New York, US
[4]National Institute of Child Health and Human Development, Office of the
Medical Director, Division for Mental Retardation, Ministry of Social
Affairs, Jerusalem, Israel
[5]Kentucky Children's Hospital, University of Kentucky,
Lexington, US

Until recently, it was thought that the adult brain is modifiable only during early stages of ontogenesis. However, neurophysiological and neuroimaging studies now indicate that the mature human brain is under certain conditions capable of substantial neuroplastic changes. The concept of plasticity is complex and can be applied to all levels of neural organization from molecular

---

[*] Correspondence: Helena Knotkova, PhD, Research Division, INBSNY, Department of Pain Medicine and Palliative Care, Beth Israel Medical Center, 120 E 16th Str., 12th fl., New York, NY, 10003, United States of America. E-mail: HKnotkov@chpnet.org

to systemic level of neural networks. Neuroplasticity reflects the ability of human brain to alter the pattern of neural activation in response to previous experience, and recent findings indicate that the effects of experience can lead to both structural as well as functional reorganization.

In the past fifteen years, advanced imaging methods have made it possible to examine how the human brain changes in response to pain, and how neuroplastic modifications of neural networks might contribute to the experience of pain. There is growing evidence indicating that chronic pain does not develop as a simple direct result of activity in nociceptive neural fibers following an initial traumatic event, but rather represents a consequence of dynamic plastic changes in sensory, affective and cognitive systems. Although relatively little is known about the physiology and chemistry underlying the neuroplasticity involved in acute- and chronic pain pathophysiology, or its reversal through treatment, the reality of these processes is now widely accepted.

Functional neuroimaging, quantitative sensory testing, neurocognitive testing and other measures substantiate the remarkable shifts in neuronal activation that may occur and correlate with clinical phenomenology, including pain perception and analgesia. The functional neural changes associated with pain include both adaptive compensatory changes, as well as maladaptive changes that may contribute to dysfunction of involved physiological systems. These findings implicate ample opportunities for pain research and pain management to explore clinical applications overarched by the phenomena of neuroplasticity in patients with chronic pain. Up to date, various approaches, such as sensory and motor training, mirror and motor imagery training, invasive- and non-invasive brain stimulation, or virtual reality and robotic applications have been explored with an ultimate goal of minimizing/preventing maladaptive neuroplastic changes and potentiating adaptive neural changes to improve function and alleviate pain in patients with various chronic pain syndromes.

Both the clinical potential of neuromodulation as well as growing knowledge on mechanisms underlying its effects are strong drivers of further translational research of enormous promise. If neuromodulatory approaches prove to be safe and effective, they could change the current view of best practice in pain management and assume a significant role in the clinic.

Chapter I

Targeting TRPV1 for pain relief

*Marcello Trevisani, PhD[1] and Arpad Szallasi, MD, PhD[*2,3]*
[1]PharmEste srl, Ferrara, Italy
[2]Departments of Pathology, Monmouth Medical Center,
Long Branch, New Jersey, US
[3]Drexel University College of Medicine,
Philadelphia, Pennsylvania, US

Preclinical research has recently uncovered new molecular mechanisms underlying the generation and transduction of pain, many of which represent opportunities for pharmacological intervention. Manipulating TRP (Transient Receptor Potential) channels on nociceptive neurons is a particularly attractive strategy in drug development in that it targets the beginning of the pain pathway. The vanilloid (capsaicin) receptor TRPV1 is a multifunctional channel involved in thermosensation (heat) and taste perception (e.g. peppers and vinegar). Importantly, TRPV1 also functions as a molecular integrator for a broad range of seemingly unrelated noxious stimuli. Indeed, TRPV1 is thought to be a major transducer of the thermal hyperalgesia that follows inflammation and/or tissue injury. Desensitization to topical TRPV1 agonists (e.g. capsaicin creams and patches) has been in clinical use for decades to alleviate chronic painful conditions like diabetic neuropathy. Currently, site-specific capsaicin and resiniferatoxin (an ultrapotent capsaicin analogue)

---

[*] Correspondence: Arpad Szallasi, MD, PhD, Department of Pathology Monmouth Medical Center, 300 Second Avenue, Long Branch, NJ 07740, United States. E-mail: aszallasi@sbhcs.com

injections are being evaluated as "molecular scalpels" to achieve permanent analgesia in cancer patients with chronic, intractable pain. In the last five years, a number of potent, small molecule TRPV1 antagonists have been advanced into clinical trials for the treatment of inflammatory, neuropathic and visceral pain. Some of these compounds have successfully passed Phase 1 safety and tolerability studies in healthy volunteers into Phase 2 studies to access efficacy in patients, whereas others showed worrisome unforeseen adverse effects (most important, hyperthermia and impaired noxious heat sensation placing the patient at risk for scalding injury) in men, prompting their withdrawal from the clinical trials. In this paper, we first give an overview of the clinical trials with TRPV1 agonists (that "reignite the fire") and then summarize the current state of the field pertaining to the known TRPV1 antagonists ("quenching the fire") in clinical development.

Introduction

Despite recent advances in our understanding of the mechanisms that cause and maintain pain, chronic pain still represents a major treatment challenge to healthcare providers. The American Pain Society estimates that at least 50 million Americans are affected by chronic pain, rendering many patients partially or totally disabled. Chronic pain already costs the country billions of dollars in health care expenses and lost productivity and the situation will certainly worsen as the population continues to age (http://www.cnn.com/ 2008/health/conditions/04/28/pain). Indeed, the neuropathic pain market in the United States is expected to double from $2.6 billion to $5 billion by 2018. Unfortunately, most analgesic drugs on the market today either provide unsatisfactory pain relief or their use is saddled by dangerous side-effects. Clearly, there is a great need for novel, potent analgesic drugs with improved safety and tolerability.

Natural products provide a window of opportunity to identify new targets for pharmacological intervention. Capsaicin, the active principle in hot chili peppers (*Capsicum annum*), is a prime example. Connoisseurs of hot spicy food are intimately familiar with the predominant pharmacological actions of capsaicin from personal experience: it induces profuse perspiration (known as gustatory sweating) as well as a hot, burning sensation that dissipates upon repeated challenge (desensitization). Capsaicin is not only a spice, however, but an extremely versatile agent whose biological uses, covered by more than 900 patents, range from culinary applications (included to improve flavor and inhibit bacterial growth) through pain killers to chemical weapons and repellants. It is still a mystery, however, why the same pungency that repels squirrels, bears or sharks is perceived as pleasurable by many human beings.

Chili pepper is extensively used in folk medicine. Some uses are time-honored and are supported by modern science whereas others are puzzling (though harmless) or have a darker side. For example, the analgesic use of capsaicin was probably independently recognized by folk healers in various cultures. In India, chili pepper tea is strongly recommended for dental pain. Native Americans traditionally rub their gums with pepper pods to relieve tooth ache. This practice also gained popularity in Europe, as was noted by the Hungarian botanist-turned-clergyman Otto Hangay in 1887 (1). As early as 1850, the Dublin Free Press recommended the use of alcoholic hot pepper extract on sore teeth (2). These early observations by astute folk healers paved the way to the on-going clinical trials with selective, small molecule TRPV1 antagonists for tooth ache and post-molar extraction pain (see below).

The modern pharmacology of capsaicin has its roots in the laboratory of Endre Högyes in Budapest, Hungary. In 1878, he made the astute observation that the capsaicin acts on sensory nerve fibers (3). However, unlike other plant products such as nicotine and atropine which attracted tremendous interest capsaicin was by and large ignored by pharmacologists until the 1950's. It was the brilliant Hungarian pharmacologist Nicholas (Miklós) Jancsó who almost single-handedly transformed capsaicin from a spice (and pharmacological oddity) to a promising analgesic drug during the tumultuous years after the 2nd World War. In 1949, he observed that "there are compounds that can selectively desensitize sensory nerve endings to noxious chemical stimuli without causing local anesthesia (4). ...Capsaicin is the paradigm of such desensitizing agents." Jancsó also postulated a central role for capsaicin-sensitive nerves in neurogenic inflammation (5).

Capsaicin was "rediscovered" in the late 1970s, as evidenced by the explosion of the literature from a few papers a year in 1977 (6, 7) to more than one a day in the late 1980s. As of today, the database of the National Library of Medicine lists 8,886 scientific papers on capsaicin. Capsaicin-containing creams (e.g. Zostrix) entered clinical practice to relieve pain associated with disease states like post-herpetic neuralgia or diabetic polyneuropathy in the 1980s. Intravesical administration of capsaicin proved beneficial in patients with overactive bladder.

In 1990 (8), the specific binding of resiniferatoxin, an ultra-potent capsaicin analogue isolated from the latex of the cactus-like perennial *E. resinifera*, furnished the first biochemical proof for the existence of the long sough-after capsaicin receptor. After this discovery, it took only seven years to clone the receptor (9), now known as TRPV1, employing an expression cloning strategy based on capsaicin-evoked Ca^{2+} uptake. The importance of TRPV1 as a pain sensor was validated by both deletion of the TRPV1 gene (10, 11) and knock-down of TRPV1 by RNA interference (12-14). Of note, TRPV1 is the founding member of the subfamily of temperature-sensitive TRP channels, the so-called "thermoTRPs". Of the 28 TRP channels discovered today, seven sense hot or warm temperatures whereas two are activated by cold. Together, these channels cover a wide temperature range with extremes that fall between 10 ^{0}C and 53 ^{0}C (15-18).

Desensitization to TRPV1 agonists (e.g. capsaicin and resiniferatoxin) is a powerful approach to relieve symptoms of nociceptive behavior in animal models of chronic pain. At present, both capsaicin-containing patches (Qutenza by Astellas Pharma, formerly NGX-4010 by NeurogesX) and site-specific, injectable capsaicin preparations (Adlea by Anesiva) are undergoing clinical trials in both oncologic and non-oncologic patient populations for the indication of chronic, intractable pain (see below). The ultrapotent capsaicin analog resiniferatoxin is moving into Phase 1 clinical trials at the National Cancer Institute as a "molecular scalpel" to disconnect pain pathways. The clinical use of TRPV1 antagonists is based on the concept that endogenous agonists ("endovanilloids") acting on TRPV1 might provide a major contribution to certain pain conditions.

Consistent with the high level of preclinical validation for TRPV1 as a pain target, many pharmaceutical companies have initiated drug screening and lead optimization programs. An array of potent and selective small molecule TRPV1 antagonists were identified, many of which are currently being evaluated in the clinic as analgesic drugs (19-36) (table 1).

Clearly, targeting TRPV1 with agonists (desensitization) and antagonists (pharmacological blockade) are two fundamentally different (complimentary rather than mutually exclusive) therapeutic approaches, both with their own specific advantages and potential adverse effects that may limit their clinical utility (table 2).

Therefore, strategies to target TRPV1 with agonists and antagonists for lasting pain relief will be discussed separately below.

Table 1. Therapeutic strategies to target TRPV1: compounds undergoing clinical trials

Compound	Company	Therapeutic indication	Development Stage (Status)	Ref
AGONISTS				
Aldea (ALGRX-4975)	Anesiva	Total knee replacement, bunionectomy	Phase III (ongoing)	[34]
Civamide (WN-1001)	Winston Laboratories	Cluster headache, osteoarthritis	Phase III (completed)	[35]
Qutenza (NGX-4010)	NeurogesX	Postherpetic neuralgia	Phase III (ongoing)	[36, 154]
ANTAGONISTS				
ABT-102	Abbott	Pain associated with inflammation, tissue injury and ischemia	Phase I (completed)	[21]
AMG-517	Amgen	Pain	Phase Ib (terminated)	[145]
AZD-1386	Astra Zeneca	Chronic nociceptive pain / GERD	Phase II (development discontinued)	[22, 24]
DWP-05195	Daewoong Pharm.	Neuropathic pain	Phase I (completed)	[26, 28]
GRC-6211	Glenmark/Lilly	Pain, migraine and urinary incontinence-associated pain and osteoarthritis.	Phase II osteoarthritis trial (suspended)	[29, 30]
JTS-653	Japan Tobaco.	Pain	Phase II (ongoing)	[31]
MK-2295	Merck/Neurogen	Pain	Discovery Phase II (completed)	[32]
PHE377	PharmEste	Neuropathic pain	Phase I (ongoing)	[33]
SB-705498	GSK	Pain, migraine, rectal pain	Phase II migraine and rectal pain (terminated) Phase II non-allergic rhinitis (intranasal) (ongoing)	[19, 25, 23]

Table 2. Targeting TRPV1 by agonists and antagonists: advantages and disadvantages

	Agonists (capsaicin)	Antagonists (small molecules)	Biological RNAi (si)RNA Antibodies
Advantages	- Sensory neurons defunctionalisation - Long lasting (weeks) effects - No/minor systemic side effect	- No induction of pain - Systemic administration - Selective effect on target	- High selectivity - Rapid development - Novel approach
Disadvantages	- Pain, neurogenic inflammation, cytotoxicity at the site of application - Require physicians - Topical/local application only - Need pre-application of local anaesthetics (lydocaine) - Unspecific effect	- No neuronal 'defunctionalisation' (weaker effect ?) - Hyperthermia - Impaired heat pain perception (to be further confirmed) - Interference with normal bladder voiding contractions (?)	- Novel approach (not well known) - May require viral delivery and/or injection

The vanilloid (capsaicin) receptor TRPV1 and nociception

Generally speaking, pain is perceived when action potentials generated in nociceptive neurons are transmitted to the somatosensory cortex. These neurons express a variety of ion channels, many of which represent potential targets for analgesic drugs (37). A subset of nociceptive neurons is distinguished by its unique sensitivity to capsaicin. In the skin, capsaicin causes an itching, pricking or burning sensation and produces cutaneous vasodilatation (flare response) and edema formation. After this initial acute neuronal excitation, a period of enhanced sensitivity to heat (thermal hyperalgesia) is established. Alternatively (after repeated challenge or when high doses are used), the previously excited neurons develop a lasting refractory state (traditionally referred to as desensitization) in which they are unresponsive not only to capsaicin but also various unrelated chemical and physical stimuli.

This capsaicin sensitivity is long considered as a functional signature of primary sensory neurons with thin-myelinated Aδ and unmyelinated C-fibers, hence the term capsaicin-sensitive afferent neurons. These neurons have somata in sensory (dorsal root, trigeminal and vagal) ganglia), reveal slow conduction capacity, and respond to noxious thermal, mechanical and chemical stimuli. The existence of a "capsaicin receptor" (now known as TRPV1) has long been anticipated based on the specific action of capsaicin on nociceptive afferent neurons and the relatively strict structure-activity requirements for capsaicin-like bioactivity (38-41).

Upon stimulation, TRPV1-expressing primary sensory neurons release a variety of pro-inflammatory neuropeptides (e.g. substance P [SP], calcitonin gene-related peptide [CGRP], and neurokinin A [NKA]) that initiate a cascade of biochemical events, globally defined as neurogenic inflammation (42). Neurogenic inflammation is thought to play a central role in the pathogenesis of various disease states that range from migraine through asthma to inflammatory bowel disease (42, 43).

TRPV1 is a polymodal receptor, sensitive to noxious heat (above 43 °C, figure 1), acidosis (pH between 5 and 6), "endovanilloids" (e.g. anandamide, arachidonic acid metabolites such as N-arachidonoyl-dopamine [NADA], 12-hydroperoxyeicosatetraenoic acid, oxidized linoleic acid metabolites, essential oils, octadecadienoids), and a variety of pungent plant products as exemplified by capsaicin (responsible for the piquancy of hot chilli peppers), resiniferatoxin (from *E. resinifera*), piperine (the pungent ingredient in black pepper), gingerol and zingerone (from ginger), camphor, as well as eugenol (a powerful essential oil found in cloves). Interestingly (and somewhat unexpectedly), TRPV1 is also activated by ethanol and venoms from jellyfish and spiders (17,44-53). In addition, TRPV1 is receptive to pro-inflammatory agents such as prostaglandins, bradykinin, adenosine triphosphate (ATP), 5-hydroxytryptamine, protease activate receptors (PAR) 1, 2 and 4, nerve growth factor (NGF) and tumor necrosis factor alpha (TNF-alpha) (54) that cause allosteric modification of the channel protein, either directly or indirectly, such that the probability of channel opening by heat, protons and capsaicin is enhanced (17, 44, 45, 55-58) (figure 1).

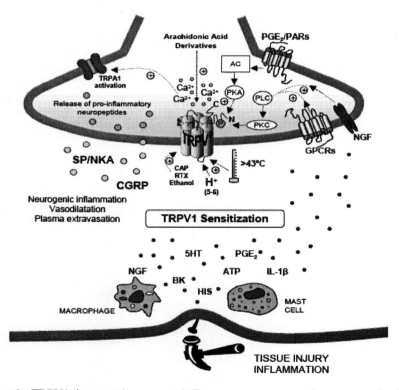

Figure 1. TRPV1 is receptive to pro-inflammatory agents such as prostaglandins, bradykinin, adenosine triphosphate (ATP), 5-hydroxytryptamine, protease activate receptors (PAR) 1, 2 and 4, nerve growth factor (NGF) and tumor necrosis factor alpha (TNF-alpha) (54) that cause allosteric modification of the channel protein, either directly or indirectly, such that the probability of channel opening by heat, protons and capsaicin is enhanced.

Thus, TRPV1 functions as a molecular integrator of painful stimuli in which each stimulus sensitizes the channel to other stimuli, with the end-result that TRPV1 acts as a molecular amplifier in the sensory neuron (59). Interestingly, TRPV1 (probably together with TRPA1) is also responsible for the paradox painful action of the commonly used general anaesthetic drug propofol (60).

Combined, these findings identify TRPV1 as a promising target to relieve inflammatory (and possibly also neuropathic and visceral) pain (figure 1). Indeed, inactivation of TRPV1 by either genetic deletion (10, 11) or pharmacological blockade experiments was reported to ameliorate heat hyperalgesia in rodent models of inflammatory pain (15-17, 61, 62).

The well-documented property of TRPV1 to become sensitized when exposed to painful stimuli has led to the hypothesis that TRPV1 is a prime contributor to the development of thermal hyperalgesia (63), which, in turn, is believed to be secondary to "peripheral sensitization" (figure 1). TRPV1 sensitization depends on several mechanisms among which phosphorylation of TRPV1 by protein kinase A (PKA), protein kinase C (PKC) and other kinases (figure 1) is of pivotal importance (55, 64-71). In fact, several inflammatory mediators (e.g. prostaglandins) enhance activation of TRPV1 by capsaicin and/or heat via a PKA-dependent pathway. Other mediators including bradykinin, NGF and anandamide were reported to increase TRPV1 activity through phospholipase C (PLC)-mediated hydrolysis of phosphatidylinositol-4,5-bisphosphate (PIP$_2$) (72). In keeping with this, it was postulated that TRPV1 is under the inhibitory control of PIP$_2$. Subsequent studies, however, reported the opposite effect (tachyphylaxis) on TRPV1 for PIP$_2$ hydrolysis. Although it has been demonstrated that PIP$_2$ could bind to both C- and N-terminus of the channel (that may provide a rational to explain differential actions), there is continuing controversy regarding the net effect of PIP$_2$ on TRPV1 (73-76).

Conversely, dephosphorylation of TRPV1 by protein phosphatases (e.g. calcineurin) promotes desensitization and represents a major mechanism of inhibitory regulation (77). Desensitization of TRPV1 to capsaicin also involves a number of intracellular components including PKA, ATP and calmodulin (74, 78-81). There appears to be a dynamic balance between phosphorylation and dephosphorylation of the TRPV1 channel that controls the activation/desensitization state of the channel (77, 82).

A clear distinction should be made between the short-lasting (seconds to minutes) desensitization of TRPV1 in channel studies and the long-lasting (up to several month) desensitization of TRPV1-expressing neurons in functional experiments. The latter phenomenon is probably better called defunctionalization, but the term "capsaicin desensitization" appears to be firmly entrenched in the literature. The mechanism of this long term "capsaicin desensitization" is poorly understood but is likely to involve changes in the expression profile of neuropeptides (e.g. SP and CGRP) and receptors (e.g. CCK receptor) involved in pain perception and processing. Combined, these changes were referred to as "vanilloid-induced messenger plasticity" (reviewed in (41)). For example, the pro-inflammatory neuropeptide SP is depleted from TRPV1-expressing neurons following capsaicin treatment whereas the expression of the endogenous analgesic peptide galanin is increased.

Regardless of the underlying mechanism, the net result is *in vivo* analgesia, a therapeutic effect that justifies continued efforts to develop site-specific capsaicin formulations for use as analgesics [reviewed in (18, 83)] (table 1 and 2) or for the treatment of urinary incontinence [reviewed in (84, 85)]. Per definition, desensitization is fully reversible. Indeed, light- or electronmicroscopic studies of tissue (skin and bladder) biopsies taken from patients undergoing capsaicin therapy revealed no evidence of neurotoxicity. Capsaicin is, however, a potential neurotoxin. In animal experiments, high ("supratherapeutic") dose capsaicin and/or resiniferatoxin administration may result in permanent nerve damage (86). Selective ablation of sensory neurons by site-specific capsaicin or resiniferatoxin injections (so-called "molecular scalpel") is an attractive approach for permanent pain relief in patients with disabling pain conditions like bone cancer pain and HIV-related poly-neuropathy.

The rationale for using potent and selective small molecule TRPV1 antagonists to relieve inflammatory pain is the concept that TRPV1 may be directly activated by agents that are present in the inflammatory soup, the so-called "endovanilloids" [reviewed in (17, 87)] (figure 1). In other words, TRPV1 antagonists are expected to prevent activation of TRPV1 by endovanilloids. Indeed, a number of agents in inflammatory soup as well as substances generated during exposure to noxious heat were implicated as potential endovanilloids. An unequivocal experimental proof for the existence of an endovanilloid responsible for inflammatory or neuropathic pain is, however, still missing.

TRPV1 knockout mice and pain-related phenotypes

During the last ten years, TRPV1 deficient mice have been extensively studied to determine the role of the receptor in normal physiological signalling and pathological processes. Two independent gene-targeting studies deleting TRPV1 alleles conclusively showed that TRPV1 is a critical channel that mediates thermal hyperalgesia under inflammatory pain conditions in mice (10, 11, 88). In addition, one study showed that TRPV1 null mice are significantly less sensitive to acute noxious heat stimulation; $TRPV1^{(-/-)}$ mice exhibited significantly larger withdrawal latencies in response to noxious heat in the hotplate assay than their wild-type littermates (10). The phenotype of the TRPV1 knockout mice generated tremendous interest in developing small molecules antagonists with an anti-hyperalgesic profile.

In wild-type mice, the endogenous fatty acid oleoylethanolamide (OEA), which is synthesized and released from the intestine upon feeding, evokes visceral pain-related behaviour. This effect was prevented by TRPV1 antagonism and was absent in $TRPV1^{(-/-)}$ mice (89). Other loss-of-function studies such as transgenic mice expressing TRPV1 shRNA (short hairpin RNA) have shown that silencing the gene encoding for TRPV1 by RNA interference significantly attenuates capsaicin-induced pain behaviour and sensitivity towards noxious heat, a similar phenotype that was observed in the TRPV1 "knockout" mice (90). Interestingly (and unlike the $TRPV1^{(-/-)}$ mice) the TRPV1 shRNA mice did not develop mechanical hypersensitivity in the spinal nerve injury model of neuropathic pain. In addition, antisense oligonucleotides and siRNAs have been reported to characterize the role of TRPV1 in pain (12-14). Surprisingly, injection of short interference RNA targeting TRPV1 significantly reduced the sensitivity of the rats to noxious heat but had no effect on the development of thermal hyperalgesia, which is highly impaired in the knockout mice. This finding may be interpreted to suggest marked species-related differences in the contribution of TRPV1 to pain states that may hinder the extrapolation of animal studies to man. An antibody directed at the extracellular loop that precedes the pore domain is an antagonist *in vitro*, but no *in vivo* characterization was reported (91).

Mice lacking a functional TRPV1 gene did not display pain behavior following intraplantar injection of phorbol 12-myristate 13-acetate (PMA), a PKC activator, suggesting that PMA-induced pain behavior was dependent on TRPV1 (88).

Taken together, these findings strongly imply TRPV1 as a pivotal polymodal receptor whose function is to combine multiple noxious physical and chemical stimuli in a nociceptive response predominantly during inflammatory conditions and tissue damage.

TRPV1 as a potential target for commonly used analgesic agents

Given the "promiscuous" nature of TRPV1 (it is activated or blocked by a broad range of chemically unrelated molecules), it is hardly surprising that TRPV1 is a potential target for a number of commonly used analgesic agents. Tramadol is a centrally-acting analgesic agent, used in treating moderate to moderately severe pain (e.g. fibromyalgia and trigeminal neuralgia). Tramadol is a synthetic codeine analogue whose therapeutic action is mainly attributed to the activation of μ-opioid receptors and to the inhibition of serotonin and norepinephrine re-uptake. In addition, tramadol was shown to inhibit the activity of voltage-dependent Na^+ channels, delayed rectifier K^+ channels, as well as γ-aminobutyric acid (GABA) type A and NMDA ionotropic receptors. Clearly, tramadol has a very complex mechanism of action which is in line with its spectrum of side-effects. Of note, tramadol is commonly combined with paracetamol/acetaminophen (e.g. Ultracet) for use in patient-controlled analgesia pumps.

Tramadol has been experimentally used in creams and gels to relieve neuropathic pain. It was recently reported that tramadol at concentrations similar to those pharmacologically active in men is capable of inducing a significant and concentration-dependent TRPV1-mediated intracellular calcium influx in CHO cells (92). On the one hand, this interaction may contribute to the analgesic action of topical tramadol preparations. On the other hand, it may explain the unexpected, capsaicin-like local side effects of tramadol creams (e.g. burning pain and erythema).

TRPV1 is also a potential target for paracetamol (acetaminophen). It was speculated that paracetamol may produce analgesia by interacting with TRPV1 expressed centrally through its metabolite N-(4-hydroxyphenyl)-5Z,8Z,11Z, 14Z -eicosatetraenamide (AM404) (93, 94).

Nefopam (Acupan) is another widely used, non-opioid, centrally-acting analgesic drug, belonging to the benzoxazocine class. The mechanism of action of nefopam is poorly understood. Multiple mechanisms appear to be involved, including blockade of TRPV1 (95). Some molecules (e.g. emodin and baicalin) commonly used to treat pain, fever or inflammatory conditions in traditional Chinese medicine (TCM) practice may, at least in part, interact with TRPV1 (96, 97).

TRPV1 agonists in pain management

Capsaicin has long been used as a topical analgesic agent to relieve chronic pain associated with postherpetic neuralgia, diabetic neuropathy and rheumatoid arthritis (18, 98, 99) (table 2). Moreover, it was recommended for musculoskeletal pains such as muscle strains and back ache. In the US, capsaicin is available as an over-the-counter (OTC) cream at concentrations of 0.075% or less under brand names like Axsain (0.025% capsaicin mixed with lidocaine) and Zostrix (0.075%). In controlled clinical trials, pain relief by these OTC capsaicin preparations proved disappointing (mostly poor and at best moderate efficacy). It was suggested that the poor efficacy of topical capsaicin creams was due to a combination of low concentration (capsaicin is absorbed poorly through human skin) at the vicinity of sensory nerve endings and patient non-compliance (capsaicin is irritant to skin when first applied and evokes violent coughing in some patients if vaporized). Indeed, low-concentration capsaicin creams probably act as counterirritants rather than true desensitizing agents. Efforts to develop capsaicin congeners with improved desensitization to irritation ratio (e.g. olvanil and nuvanil) (100) met with limited success. To circumvent these problems, high-concentration capsaicin preparations like occlusive patches and site-specific injections were developed that are detailed below.

Capsaicin formulations in clinical development

1) Anesiva (http://www.anesiva.com) is developing Adlea™ (formerly ALGRX-4975) as a site-specific, injectable preparation of capsaicin for the potential management of pain associated with osteoarthritis (OA), tendonitis and postsurgical conditions, as well as for neuropathic pain occurring secondary to nerve injury. Anesiva disclosed the outcome of its ACTIVE-2 (Assessment of highly purified Capsaicin to ImproVE pain) trial in 2009. The ACTIVE-2 trial enrolled 217 patients undergoing total knee arthroplasty in multiple orthopaedic surgery centres who were randomized to receive either a

single 60 ml dose of Adlea (0.25 mg/ml capsaicin) or placebo instilled into the surgical site. The primary endpoint of the study (post-operative pain in the 4 to 48 hour period, determined as the area under the NPRS curve) was reported as statistically significant (p=0.03). The study also met its secondary endpoint by a statistically significant reduction in opioid consumption.

In the ACTIVE-1 trial, ALGRX-4975 (4 ml of 0.25 mg/ml) was reported to significantly reduce the mean VAS pain scores at 8 h and 24 h post unilateral bunionectomy after a single intra-operative instillation (101). ALGRX-4975 (0.5 ml of 0.2 mg/ml) also produced a significant reduction in pain in patients with intermetatarsal neuroma at week 1 and 4 compared to placebo (102). Furthermore, ALGRX-4975 significantly reduced pain scores and improved grip strength in patients with lateral epicondylitis (103) and lowered WOMAC (Western Ontario McMasters OA index) pain scores in patients with end-stage OA of the knee waiting for knee replacement (101). From baseline to 8 weeks, patients in all Adlea treatment groups reported large reductions in WOMAC pain scores. During inguinal hernia repair, intraoperative instillation of ALGRX-4975 (15 ml of 0.067 mg/ml) significantly improved analgesia relative to placebo during the first 3–4 days following surgery (104). However, a study with patients undergoing open cholecystectomy found no difference in average pain scores between treated and placebo groups.

2) Winston Laboratories (http://www.winstonlabs.com) is developing Civamide, a synthetic isomer (*cis*) of capsaicin. Civamide (50 μg) given intranasally was reported to significantly reduce episodic cluster headache (105, 106). Moreover, a single dose of either 20 μg or 150 μg of Civamide demonstrated clinical efficacy against single migraine headache, with or without aura (106). As per the clinicaltrials.gov website, three Phase 3 studies of Civamide have been completed, two in cluster headache and one in osteoarthritis of the knee (107). The results of these trials are yet to be made public.

3) Qutenza^{TM} (formerly, NGX-4010) is a rapid delivery dermal patch application system containing high-concentrations (8% w/w) of synthetic (*trans*) capsaicin for sustained pain relief. The patch was originally developed by Neuroges-X (www.neurogesx.com) and is now marketed in Europe by Astellas Pharma for the management of neuropathic pain due to postherpetic neuralgia (PHN). A randomized, two-arm, double-blind, multicenter Phase 3 clinical trial involving 402 patients was conducted to evaluate the efficacy and safety of a single 60 minute application of NGX-4010 in patients with PHN (108). In this study, the control (placebo) patch contained a low (0.04%)

concentration of capsaicin to cause a mild burning sensation (otherwise patients could easily make a distinction between NGX-4010 and placebo). The results showed a significant (p=0.001) ~30% reduction in pain (determined by the Numerical Pain Rating Scale, NPRS) compared to placebo (19%) during the duration of the study (up to 8 weeks). Forty-two percent of patients responded to the treatment with a reduction in NPRS score of at least 30% versus 25% in the control group. On the Patient Global Impression of Change scale, a slight majority (53%) of patients rated themselves improved at week 8 versus 42% in the control group. In a second Phase 3, confirmatory trial involving 416 patients in the US and Canada, the NGX-4010 group demonstrated a 32% reduction in pain from baseline compared to a 24% decrease in the placebo group (109, 110). Importantly, the long-term use of NGX-4010 was well-tolerated without any evidence of cumulative toxicity.

NGX-4010 (single application) was also evaluated in patients with moderate to severe pain due to HIV-associated distal sensory polyneuropathy (HIV-DSP) (111). A total of 307 patients were randomized and treated at 30 Pain Clinics in the US. NGX-4010 provided a lasting (12 weeks) reduction in pain by 23% on the standard NPRS versus 10.7% in the control group. A 40 week open-label extension study demonstrated consistent pain relief over the entire study period; the magnitude of the response was similar to that seen in the 12-weeks controlled study. A second, Phase 3 trial was conducted to confirm the results of the first trial. In the second trial, however, pain relief did not reach statistical significance (110, 112).

An open-label, multicenter clinical study with 91 patients was completed to evaluate the efficacy of NGX-4010 for painful diabetic neuropathy. The results showed a mean decrease of 32% in pain scores from baseline during weeks 2 to 12 (113).

TRPV1 antagonists:
A pre-clinical overview

The first competitive TRPV1 antagonist, capsazepine, was developed by starting from the capsaicin structure (114). Though extremely useful in the research laboratory, capsazepine was a poor clinical candidate. Most important, capsazepine is not selective for TRPV1; in fact, it inhibits nicotinic and voltage-gated calcium channels [reviewed in (17, 41)], as well as TRPM8 (115, 116).

Following the molecular cloning of TRPV1, most major pharmaceutical companies (as well as many small biotech companies) have initiated drug screening and lead optimisation programs to identify potent small-molecule TRPV1 antagonists for the treatment of different pain states. These efforts have resulted in the identification of a large (and still growing) number of potent and efficacious TRPV1 antagonists [see table 2; reviewed in (16, 61, 62, 117)]. As discussed above, TRPV1 is a polymodal receptor activated by multiple stimuli that interact with different domains of the channel protein. Not unexpectedly, some TRPV1 blockers turned out to be stimulus-specific whereas others appear to block several means of activation (118, 119). For instance, AMG0610 (from Amgen) and SB-366791 (developed by GlaxoSmithKline) inhibit the activation of rat TRPV1 by capsaicin but not by acid, whereas I-RTX, BCTC, AMG6880, AMG7472, AMG9810 and A-425619 are TRPV1 antagonists that do not differentiate between capsaicin and protons (118, 120-122). Compounds were also identified (e.g. AMG8562) that do not block heat-evoked activation of rat TRPV1 (119).

Importantly, there are species-related differences in the stimulus selectivity of TRPV1 blockers. For instance, capsazepine and SB-366791 are more effective in blocking proton-induced gating of human TRPV1 than of rat TRPV1 (118, 123), whereas AMG8562 antagonizes heat activation of human but not rat TRPV1 (119). Of these inhibitors, I-RTX, the urea analog BCTC and the cinnamide analog SB-366791 are the best studied. Within this group, I-RTX and SB-366791 are quite selective versus other receptors and channels, whereas BCTC (similarly to capsazepine) is also a good inhibitor of TRPM8 (124).

Several structurally different TRPV1 antagonists such as capsazepine, BCTC, A-425619 (Abbott), A-784168, GRC-6211 (Glenmark), PHE377 (PharmEste) and the quinazolinone "Compound 26" are reported to decrease hypersensitivity in rat neuropathic pain models (29, 30, 125-132).

The recently disclosed TRPV1 receptor antagonist from Abbott, ABT-102 (table 2) which is currently undergoing a Phase 1 clinical trial, exhibits analgesic properties in several rodent pain models, including chronic inflammatory, bone cancer, and postoperative pain. Another Abbott molecule (ABT-116) exhibited potent *in vitro* and *in vivo* activity, possessing a suitable profile for advancement to clinical development for pain management (21, 133-135). Compound A-995662 exhibited anti-pain effect in a model of rat knee joint pain partly by reducing the release of glutamate and CGRP from the spinal cord (136).

It should be mentioned here that preclinical models of pain may result in an underestimation of the clinical utility of TRPV1 antagonist because they do not adequately address the extent of spontaneous or ongoing pain (137). It is also worth noting that while pain due to cancer may only partly arise from neuropathy, TRPV1 antagonists have exhibited effectiveness in models of cancer pain (138, 139).

TRPV1 and body temperature regulation

Activation of TRPV1 by capsaicin is known to transiently decrease body temperature in various species, including man. Indeed, this hypothermic response was extensively used to quantify capsaicin-like bioactivity. The hypothermic response was attributed to a combination of increased heat loss (skin vasodilation in animals and gustatory sweating in man) and reduced heat production (41, 140). It was postulated that capsaicin alters the thermosensitivity of preoptic heat sensors, thereby tricking the animals to believe that they feel hot. Indeed, capsaicin microinjected into the preoptic area mimicked the hypothermic action of systemic capsaicin administration and morphological alteration similar to those seen in sensory ganglia was detected in preoptic area neurons. Interestingly, animals desensitized to capsaicin lose their ability to regulate their core temperature: when placed in hot environment, such animals suffer heat stroke. Nonetheless, capsaicin-desensitized animals display normal body temperature when kept in ambient temperature environment. Therefore, it was somewhat unexpected that some, but not all, TRPV1 antagonists paradoxically cause hyperthermia in several species including man (129, 141, 142).

The question which still remains to be answered unequivocally is whether the hyperthermic action of TRPV1 antagonists is "on-target", that is un-separable from their analgesic action. The findings are confusing. TRPV1 $^{(-/-)}$ mice have an apparently normal body temperature and rats whose TRPV1-expressing neurons have been ablated by high-dose neonatal capsaicin administration do not show hyperthermia either. The hyperthermic action of some TRPV1 antagonists was first reported in 2006 at the Spring Pain Conference, Cayman Islands. It was noted that the increase in body temperature was moderate ($\sim$0.5 ^{0}C); it could be mitigated by common antipyretic drugs like acetaminophen; and it disappeared ("desensitized") upon repeated administration. It was, however, worrisome that the febrile reaction was exacerbated in animals exposed to bacterial endotoxins (LPS).

In 2008, Amgen announced the early termination of a Phase 1b dental pain (molar extraction) study with their clinical candidate molecule, AMG517, because it caused a lasting (1-4 days) marked hyperthermia response (up to 40.2 ^{0}C) in human volunteers. This finding provided the experimental foundation for the concept [most recently refuted by Romanovsky and colleagues, (143)] that the predominant function of TRPV1 is body temperature regulation (144). It was postulated that TRPV1 has an endogenous tone which is important for the maintenance of normal body temperature (142, 145). If this tone is increased (for example by administering the exogenous agonist capsaicin), core temperature starts dropping. Conversely, decreasing the tone by TRPV1 antagonists leads to hyperthermia. This simple model is, however, inconsistent with the experimental findings. The hypothermic activity of capsaicin has been firmly linked to the preoptic area. Capsaicin when microinjected into this brain nucleus is causing a marked hypothermic response. By contrast, the low CNS penetrant TRPV1 antagonist, AMG0347, is not more effective in causing hyperthermia when administered into the brain (intracerebroventricularly) or spinal cord (intrathecally) than when given systemically (intravenously) (146). This observation was interpreted to imply that TRPV1 expressed on a peripheral site mediates the effect of TRPV1 antagonist on core body temperature. In other words, the sites that are responsible for the hypothermic activity of capsaicin (preoptic area) and hyperthermic action of TRPV1 antagonists are anatomically distinct. The site that mediates the febrile reaction of the antagonists is now believed to be in the abdomen, probably the GI tract (though this concept has been questioned recently) (146).

Several strategies were tried to mitigate the hyperthermic action of TRPV1 antagonists. Similar to agonist-induced hypothermia that disappears after repeated administration, antagonist-induced hyperthermia also shows attenuation after repeated dosing (147). It was suggested that the initial hyperthermia can be adequately managed by common antipyretic agents like acetaminophen. A more attractive approach is to eliminate the undesirable side-effect of TRPV1 antagonists on thermoregulation by chemical modification of the pharmacophore.

In the rat, it was feasible to eliminate hyperthermia while preserving antihyperalgesia by differential modulation of distinct modes of TRPV1 activation. Compounds (e.g. AMG8562) that prevented the activation of rat TRPV1 by capsaicin, but not by low pH (referred to as Profile C antagonists), had no effect on body temperature (119).

Unfortunately, the observations made in rats did not hold true in dogs, indicating that it would be very problematic to extrapolate results to humans.

Importantly, at least two potent TRPV1 antagonists (GRC6211 and PHE377) appear to be devoid of any febrile reaction when administered to rodents or dogs. At present, there is no mechanistic explanation why some TRPV1 antagonists elevate body temperature whereas others do not.

TRPV1 antagonists and noxious heat perception in humans

In keeping with its function as a noxious heat sensor, an impaired detection of painful heat was described in TRPV1 knockout mice (10). Moreover, TRPV1 antagonists were reported to elevate the withdrawal reflex threshold in response to noxious heat in preclinical species (148-150).

Most recently, clinical studies have confirmed the role of TRPV1 as a noxious heat sensor in humans demonstrating the involvement of the channel in heat perception in healthy volunteers. Indeed, heat pain threshold was significantly elevated in non-sensitized skin of healthy volunteers following 400 mg SB-705498 (*GlaxoSmithKline*) oral administration (19, 151). Subsequently, investigators at Merck-Neurogen have reported that compound MK-2295 markedly blunted heat perception in healthy human subjects (quantitative thermal sensory tests, pain evoked by hand immersion into or sipping hot water) with no sign of tachyphylaxis (150, 152). Similar results were observed by AstraZeneca with the TRPV1 antagonist, AZD1386. AZD1386 was investigated in two Phase 1 trials in healthy volunteers and found to increase mean thresholds for heat-induced pain (151). Interestingly, the enhancement in heat pain threshold persisted after repeated dosing of compound AZD1386.

The enhanced heat pain threshold and tolerance induced by TRPV1 antagonists in healthy volunteers (which is apparently greater than those observed in pre-clinical species) is worrisome for its potential to cause scalding injury. Indeed, some subjects taking MK-2295 perceived potentially harmful temperatures as innocuous. These individuals could have suffered scalding injuries when taking hot shower or drinking hot coffee. Importantly, the effect of TRPV1 antagonists on heat pain sensation does not attenuate after multiple dosages.

TRPV1 antagonist undergoing clinical trials

Several small molecule TRPV1 antagonists are currently undergoing Phase 1 and 2 clinical trials for indications related to pain (table 2).

GlaxoSmithKline disclosed its Phase 1 results obtained with SB-705498. SB-705498 is a selective and potent TRPV1 antagonist that blocks channel activation by capsaicin, protons and heat with similar potencies (IC_{50} values are 3 nM, 6 nM, and 7 nM, respectively). In the first part of the study, single doses of SB-705498 ranging from 2 to 200 mg did not display efficacy in the capsaicin-evoked flare test (19). However, in the second part of the study, a single oral dose of 400 mg SB-705498 substantially reduced pain from cutaneous capsaicin challenge (0.075% capsaicin cream applied to the forearm) compared to placebo. Importantly, SB-705498 did not show any serious adverse effects in the study. The effect of *per os* SB-705495 on dermal heat sensitivity following capsaicin or UVB challenge was also evaluated. In these studies, two important observations were made. First, SB-705498 caused a modest, but significant, increase in noxious heat perception threshold (up to 1.3 ^{0}C). Second, SB-705498 prevented thermal hyperalgesia caused by UVB, but not capsaicin, treatment. This is very surprising and puzzling since the occupation of TRPV1 by SB-705498 was expected to prevent capsaicin binding to the channel and the resultant capsaicin-induced thermal hyperalgesia. It should be remembered, however, that SB-705498 did only reduce, but did not eliminate, the flare response to capsaicin. Thus, one might speculate that "endovanilloids" generated during the residual inflammatory response have sensitized the channel to heat. In December 2005, an active-controlled, placebo-controlled, randomized, single-blind, Phase 2 trial (NCT00281684, VRA105345) was initiated in subjects with dental pain following third molar tooth extraction. The subjects were to receive a single oral dose of SB-705498, placebo or co-codamol. The study was completed by February 2008 and no results have been revealed, yet (25).

Abbott is developing a tablet formulation of ABT-102 for the potential treatment of pain associated with tissue injury, inflammation and ischemia. A phase I assessment has been recently completed (21).

A Phase 2 trial with GRC-6211 (Glenmark-Eli Lilly) for ostheoarthritic pain was suspended due to undisclosed reasons. Additional indications include incontinence and neuropathic pain (29, 30).

Merck was developing MK-2295 (NGD-8243; MRK-2295) for the potential treatment of pain and cough. As discussed above, MK-2295 has markedly increased the noxious heat pain threshold in humans, placing the study participants at the risk of scalding injury. For example, only 66% of individuals on 25 mg of MK-2295 found sipped 70 ^{0}C water too hot for rapid consumption compared to every person in the control group. These findings question the clinical safety of MK-2295 (and maybe all TRPV1 antagonists) (32). In 2009, MK-2295 was disclosed to be in preclinical development.

Japan Tobacco is developing an oral TRPV1 antagonist, namely JTS-653, for the potential treatment of pain and overactive bladder. By July 2010, the compound was in phase II trials (153).

Compound PHE377 (33), a potent TRPV1 antagonist developed by PharmEste to treat diabetic neuropathic pain and post herpetic neuralgia, is currently undergoing a Phase 1 clinical trial.

Daewoong Pharmaceutical is developing DWP-05195, a TRPV1 antagonist, for the potential treatment of neuropathic pain. By February 2009, a phase I trial had begun (26, 28).

AstraZeneca was developing AZD-1386, an oral solution formulation of a TRPV1 antagonist for the potential treatment of gastroesophageal reflux disease (GERD). However, in January 2011, AstraZeneca discontinued the development of AZD-1386 (22). In April 2008, an active-controlled, placebo-controlled, randomized, double-blind phase 2 trial (NCT00672646, D5090C00010) was initiated in subjects with pain due to third molar extraction. AZD-1386 (55 mg *per os*) caused significant pain relief. The drug was well-tolerated though a modest increase in body temperature (~0.4 ^{0}C in average) was noticed in most patients, exceeding 38 ^{0}C in one individual (24).

Conclusions

The discovery of TRP channels in nociceptive neurons has spawned extensive research efforts to understand the role of these channels in the initiation and maintenance of pain conditions and to identify potent and selective small molecule antagonists that can be exploited for therapeutic purposes (reviewed in 17). Since these channels are strategically located at the periphery where the pain pathway begins, it is hoped that TRP antagonists will be devoid of the side-effects that plague the clinical use of centrally-acting analgesic agents. Of TRP channels that are present in nociceptive neurons, the vanilloid (capsaicin) receptor TRPV1 has attracted the most attention so far due to the well-documented clinical potential of capsaicin to relieve pain (that predates the molecular cloning of TRPV1) and the ample preclinical evidence accumulated recently suggesting that TRPV1 antagonists can also provide benefit to patients (15, 18, 20, 61).

Desensitization to capsaicin is a unique approach to lasting pain relief. After an initial excitatory response (that can be minimized by topical analgesic agents like lidocaine), TRPV1-expressing neurons develop a long-lasting (weeks in animal experiments and several months in clinical studies) refractory state in which the neurons are silent regardless of the nature of the noxious stimulus (40-42). This is important since capsaicin-sensitive neurons express a broad range of channels (from sodium channels [e.g. Nav1.8] through TRP channels to acid-sensitive ASICs) that are involved in pain perception. All of these channels are silent during capsaicin desensitization. Desensitization to systemic capsaicin (or its ultrapotent analogue, resiniferatoxin) administration is an extremely powerful approach to mitigate pain in animal models. For example, resiniferatoxin by means of a single s.c. injection (100 µg/kg) can completely prevent and/or cure pain behavior in the Bennett model of neuropathic pain (G. Bennett, M. Tal, A. Szallasi, unpublished observations).

Systemic desensitization is, however, not feasible in human patients for fear of potentially fatal side-effects (e.g. respiratory arrest) if capsaicin is inadvertently injected into the circulation. In controlled clinical trials, capsaicin-containing creams gave disappointing results due to a combination of limited efficacy and poor patient compliance (reviewed in 18). To circumvent these problems, occlusive high capsaicin concentration patches (e.g. Qutenza) and site-specific capsaicin injections (e.g. Adlea) were developed (83, 110). In clinical trials, Qutenza showed significant pain relief compared to placebo in patients with PHN (reviewed in 100). Importantly, Qutenza was devoid of any serious side-effect, inclusive body temperature regulation.

TRPV1 antagonists offer a novel mechanism of action for the potential treatment of a wide range of painful conditions. The pharmaceutical industry showed great success in the identification and development of potent small molecule TRPV1 antagonist candidates (reviewed 20). At least twelve compounds entered Phase 1 clinical testing and five of these agents have progressed into Phase 2 'proof-of-concept' studies. The results of these trials are keenly awaited. If the promise of these compounds from preclinical and Phase 1 work is confirmed by the proof-of-concept studies, TRPV1 antagonists may represent the first mechanistically novel class of analgesic drugs for many years. The high expectations, however, were recently replaced by cautious optimism. The key issues with some TRPV1 antagonists are hyperthermia (e.g. AMG517) and a potential for scalding injury (e.g. MK-2295) due to impaired noxious heat detection (144, 152). However, not all TRPV1 antagonists are created equal and a better understanding of the gating mechanisms of the channel might aid us in selecting future antagonists that are better tolerated. Further clinical trials are needed to assess the likely risk/benefit profile for patients with various painful conditions.

In summary, desensitization of capsaicin-sensitive neurons by agonists and pharmacological blockade of TRPV1 by antagonists are two fundamentally different and complimentary therapeutic approaches for pain relief. Only localized pain is amenable to topical and/or site-specific capsaicin therapy. By contrast, small molecule TRPV1 antagonists may be administered *per* os to alleviate more generalized pain. The balance between the beneficial actions and adverse effects of TRPV1 antagonists must be carefully and pragmatically evaluated in order to determine if these drugs could emerge as the next generation of pain killers. Regardless of the outcome, the tremendous experience obtained with therapeutic targeting of the TRPV1 receptor should greatly facilitate on-going efforts to capitalize on the additional TRP channels (e.g. TRPA1, TRPV3 and TRPM8) that are present in nociceptive neurons.

References

Hangay O. A Paprikáról, Tekintettel a Régi Füszerekre (On peppers, with special regard to old spices). Szammeb Imre Nyomdája, Székes-Fehérvár; 1887.

Turnbull A. Tincture of capsaicin as a remedy for chilblains and toothache. Dublin Free Press 1850;1:95–6.

Högyes E. Beitrage zur physiologischen wirkung der bestandteile des Capsicum annum. Arch Exp Pathol Pharmakol 1878;9:117–30.

Jancsó NA. Desensitization of sensory nerve endings. Kísérletes Orvostudomány 1949;2(2 (Suppl)):15.

Jancso N, Jancso-Gabor A, Szolcsanyi J. Direct evidence for neurogenic inflammation and its prevention by denervation and by pretreatment with capsaicin. Br J Pharmacol Chemother 1967;31(1):138-51.

Jancso G, Kiraly E, Jancso-Gabor A. Pharmacologically induced selective degeneration of chemosensitive primary sensory neurones. Nature 1977;270(5639):741-43.

Szolcsanyi J. A pharmacological approach to elucidation of the role of different nerve fibres and receptor endings in mediation of pain. J Physiol (Paris), in press.

Szallasi A, Blumberg PM. Resiniferatoxin, a phorbol-related diterpene, acts as an ultrapotent analog of capsaicin, the irritant constituent in red pepper. Neuroscience 1989;30(2):515-20.

Caterina MJ, Schumacher MA, Tominaga M, Rosen TA, Levine JD, Julius D. The capsaicin receptor: a heat-activated ion channel in the pain pathway. Nature 1997;389(6653):816-24.

Caterina MJ, Leffler A, Malmberg AB, Martin WJ, Trafton J, Petersen-Zeitz KR, et al. Impaired nociception and pain sensation in mice lacking the capsaicin receptor. Science 2000;288(5464):306-13.

Davis JB, Gray J, Gunthorpe MJ, Hatcher JP, Davey PT, Overend P, et al. Vanilloid receptor-1 is essential for inflammatory thermal hyperalgesia. Nature 2000;405(6783):183-7.

Christoph T, Gillen C, Mika J, Grunweller A, Schafer MK, Schiene K, et al. Antinociceptive effect of antisense oligonucleotides against the vanilloid receptor VR1/TRPV1. Neurochem Int 2007;50(1):281-90.

Christoph T, Grunweller A, Mika J, Schafer MK, Wade EJ, Weihe E, et al. Silencing of vanilloid receptor TRPV1 by RNAi reduces neuropathic and visceral pain in vivo. Biochem Biophys Res Commun 2006;350(1):238-43.

Kasama S, Kawakubo M, Suzuki T, Nishizawa T, Ishida A, Nakayama J. RNA interference-mediated knock-down of transient receptor potential vanilloid 1 prevents forepaw inflammatory hyperalgesia in rat. Eur J Neurosci 2007;25(10):2956-63.

Malmberg A, Bley K. Turning up the Heat on Pain: TRPV1 Receptors in Pain and Inflammation. Birkhäuser, Basel, Switzerland 2005.

Roberts LA, Connor M. TRPV1 antagonists as a potential treatment for hyperalgesia. Recent Patents CNS Drug Discov 2006;1(1):65-76.

Szallasi A, Cortright DN, Blum CA, Eid SR. The vanilloid receptor TRPV1: 10 years from channel cloning to antagonist proof-of-concept. Nat Rev Drug Discov 2007;6(5):357-72.

Knotkova H, Pappagallo M, Szallasi A. Capsaicin (TRPV1 Agonist) therapy for pain relief: farewell or revival? Clin J Pain 2008;24(2):142-54.

Chizh BA, O'Donnell MB, Napolitano A, Wang J, Brooke AC, Aylott MC, et al. The effects of the TRPV1 antagonist SB-705498 on TRPV1 receptor-mediated activity and inflammatory hyperalgesia in humans. Pain 2007;132(1-2):132-41.

Faltynek C, Gomtsyan A. Vanilloid receptor TRPV1 in drug discovery: targeting pain and other pathological disorders. John Wiley, 2009.

http://clinicaltrials.gov/ct2/results?term=ABT-102.

http://www.astrazeneca.com/cs/Satellite?blobcol=urldataandblobheader=application%2Fpdf andblobheadername1=Content-Dispositionandblobheadername2=MDT-Typeandblobheadervalue1=inline%3B+filename%3DDownload-pipeline-summary.pdfandblobheadervalue2=abinary%3B+charset%3DUTF-8andblobkey=idandblobtable=MungoBlobsandblobwhere=1285619440126andssbina ry=true

http://www.gsk.com/investors/product_pipeline/docs/GSK-product-pipeline-Feb-2010.pdf.

http://clinicaltrials.gov/ct2/results?term=AZD-1386.

http://clinicaltrials.gov/ct2/show/NCT00281684?cond.

http://clinicaltrials.gov/ct2/show/NCT00969787?term=05195andrank=1.

http://www.clinicaltrials.gov/ct2/show/NCT00387140?

http://www.daewoong.com

http://www.glenmarkpharma.com/media/pdf/releases/GRC_6211.pdf.

http://www.glenmarkpharma.com/research/clinical.html.

http://www.jt.com/investors/results/pharmaceuticals/pdf/P.L.20100729_E.pdf.

http://www.neurogen.com/index.php?option=com_contentandview=articleandid=47andIte
mid=2andphpMyAdmin=34a2390c0eecf801a871d79668695b95.

http://www.pharmeste.com/include/PHE377.pdf.

http://clinicaltrials.gov/ct2/results?term=ALGRX-4975.

http://clinicaltrials.gov/ct2/results?term=civamide.

http://clinicaltrials.gov/ct2/results?term=NGX-4010.

Nilius B, Owsianik G, Voets T, Peters JA. Transient receptor potential cation channels in disease. Physiol Rev 2007;87(1):165-217.

Szolcsanyi J, Bartho L. Capsaicin-sensitive non-cholinergic excitatory innervation of the guinea-pig tracheobronchial smooth muscle. Neurosci Lett 1982;34(3):247-51.

Maggi CA, Meli A. The sensory-efferent function of capsaicin-sensitive sensory neurons. Gen Pharmacol 1988;19(1):1-43.

Holzer P. Capsaicin: cellular targets, mechanisms of action, and selectivity for thin sensory neurons. Pharmacol Rev 1991;43(2):143-201.

Szallasi A, Blumberg PM. Vanilloid (Capsaicin) receptors and mechanisms. Pharmacol Rev 1999;51(2):159-212.

Geppetti P, Holzer P. Neurogenic inflammation. Boca Raton: CRC Press; 1996.

Butler CA, Heaney LG. Neurogenic inflammation and asthma. Inflamm Allergy Drug Targets 2007;6(2):127-32.

Caterina MJ, Julius D. The vanilloid receptor: a molecular gateway to the pain pathway. Annu Rev Neurosci 2001;24:487-517.

Trevisani M, Smart D, Gunthorpe MJ, Tognetto M, Barbieri M, Campi B, et al. Ethanol elicits and potentiates nociceptor responses via the vanilloid receptor-1. Nat Neurosci 2002;5(6):546-51.

Patapoutian A, Peier AM, Story GM, Viswanath V. ThermoTRP channels and beyond: mechanisms of temperature sensation. Nat Rev Neurosci 2003;4(7):529-39.

Siemens J, Zhou S, Piskorowski R, Nikai T, Lumpkin EA, Basbaum AI, et al. Spider toxins activate the capsaicin receptor to produce inflammatory pain. Nature 2006;444(7116):208-12.

Cromer BA, McIntyre P. Painful toxins acting at TRPV1. Toxicon 2008;51(2):163-73.

Pingle SC, Matta JA, Ahern GP. Capsaicin receptor: TRPV1 a promiscuous TRP channel. Handb Exp Pharmacol 2007(179):155-71.

Ohkawara S, Tanaka-Kagawa T, Furukawa Y, Nishimura T, Jinno H. Activation of the human transient receptor potential vanilloid subtype 1 by essential oils. Biol Pharm Bull 2010;33(8):1434-7.

Flores CM, Vasko MR. The deorphanization of TRPV1 and the emergence of octadecadienoids as a new class of lipid transmitters. Mol Interv. 2010;10(3):137-40.

Bohlen CJ, Priel A, Zhou S, King D, Siemens J, Julius D. A bivalent tarantula toxin activates the capsaicin receptor, TRPV1, by targeting the outer pore domain. Cell 2010;141(5):834-45.

Patwardhan AM, Akopian AN, Ruparel NB, Diogenes A, Weintraub ST, Uhlson C, et al. Heat generates oxidized linoleic acid metabolites that activate TRPV1 and produce pain in rodents. J Clin Invest 2010;120(5):1617-26.

Spicarova D, Palecek J. Tumor necrosis factor alpha sensitizes spinal cord TRPV1 receptors to the endogenous agonist N-oleoyldopamine. J Neuroinflammation 2010;7:49.

Vellani V, Mapplebeck S, Moriondo A, Davis JB, McNaughton PA. Protein kinase C activation potentiates gating of the vanilloid receptor VR1 by capsaicin, protons, heat and anandamide. J Physiol 2001;534(Pt 3):813-25.

Amadesi S, Nie J, Vergnolle N, Cottrell GS, Grady EF, Trevisani M, et al. Protease-activated receptor 2 sensitizes the capsaicin receptor transient receptor potential vanilloid receptor 1 to induce hyperalgesia. J Neurosci 2004;24(18):4300-12.

Vellani V, Kinsey AM, Prandini M, Hechtfischer SC, Reeh P, Magherini PC, et al. Protease activated receptors 1 and 4 sensitize TRPV1 in nociceptive neurones. Mol Pain 2010;6(1):61.

Gunthorpe MJ, Benham CD, Randall A, Davis JB. The diversity in the vanilloid (TRPV) receptor family of ion channels. Trends Pharmacol Sci 2002;23(4):183-91.

Crandall M, Kwash J, Yu W, White G. Activation of protein kinase C sensitizes human VR1 to capsaicin and to moderate decreases in pH at physiological temperatures in Xenopus oocytes. Pain 2002;98(1-2):109-17.

Fischer MJ, Leffler A, Niedermirtl F, Kistner K, Eberhardt M, Reeh PW, et al. The General Anesthetic Propofol Excites Nociceptors by Activating Trpv1 and Trpa1 Rather Than Gabaa Receptors. J Biol Chem 2010; [Epub ahead of print].

Gunthorpe MJ, Szallasi A. Peripheral TRPV1 receptors as targets for drug development: new molecules and mechanisms. Curr Pharm De. 2008;14(1):32-41.

Gharat L, Szallasi A. Advances in the design and therapeutic use of capsaicin receptor TRPV1 agonists and antagonists. Expert Opin Ther Patents 2008;18:159-209.

Reeh PW, Petho G. Nociceptor excitation by thermal sensitization--a hypothesis. Prog Brain Res 2000;129:39-50.

Premkumar LS, Ahern GP. Induction of vanilloid receptor channel activity by protein kinase C. Nature 2000;408(6815):985-990.

Tominaga M, Wada M, Masu M. Potentiation of capsaicin receptor activity by metabotropic ATP receptors as a possible mechanism for ATP-evoked pain and hyperalgesia. Proc Natl Acad Sci USA 2001;98(12):6951-56.

Kagaya M, Lamb J, Robbins J, Page CP, Spina D. Characterization of the anandamide induced depolarization of guinea-pig isolated vagus nerve. Br J Pharmacol 2002;137(1):39-48.

Olah Z, Karai L, Iadarola MJ. Protein kinase C(alpha) is required for vanilloid receptor 1 activation. Evidence for multiple signaling pathways. J Biol Chem 2002;277(38):35752-59.

Bhave G, Hu HJ, Glauner KS, Zhu W, Wang H, Brasier DJ, et al. Protein kinase C phosphorylation sensitizes but does not activate the capsaicin receptor transient receptor potential vanilloid 1 (TRPV1). Proc Natl Acad Sci USA 2003;100(21):12480-85.

Varga A, Bolcskei K, Szoke E, Almasi R, Czeh G, Szolcsanyi J, et al. Relative roles of protein kinase A and protein kinase C in modulation of transient receptor potential vanilloid type 1 receptor responsiveness in rat sensory neurons in vitro and peripheral nociceptors in vivo. Neuroscience 2006;140(2):645-57.

Vetter I, Wyse BD, Monteith GR, Roberts-Thomson SJ, Cabot PJ. The mu opioid agonist morphine modulates potentiation of capsaicin-evoked TRPV1 responses through a cyclic AMP-dependent protein kinase A pathway. Mol Pain 2006;2:22.

Zhang X, McNaughton PA. Why pain gets worse: the mechanism of heat hyperalgesia. J Gen Physiol 2006;128(5):491-3.

Prescott ED, Julius D. A modular PIP2 binding site as a determinant of capsaicin receptor sensitivity. Science 2003;300(5623):1284-8.

Brauchi S, Orta G, Mascayano C, Salazar M, Raddatz N, Urbina H, et al. Dissection of the components for PIP2 activation and thermosensation in TRP channels. Proc Natl Acad Sci USA 2007;104(24):10246-51.

Lishko PV, Procko E, Jin X, Phelps CB, Gaudet R. The ankyrin repeats of TRPV1 bind multiple ligands and modulate channel sensitivity. Neuron 2007;54(6):905-18.

Stein AT, Ufret-Vincenty CA, Hua L, Santana LF, Gordon SE. Phosphoinositide 3-kinase binds to TRPV1 and mediates NGF-stimulated TRPV1 trafficking to the plasma membrane. J Gen Physiol 2006;128(5):509-22.

Lukacs V, Thyagarajan B, Varnai P, Balla A, Balla T, Rohacs T. Dual regulation of TRPV1 by phosphoinositides. J Neurosci 2007;27(26):7070-80.

Mohapatra DP, Nau C. Regulation of Ca2+-dependent desensitization in the vanilloid receptor TRPV1 by calcineurin and cAMP-dependent protein kinase. J Biol Chem 2005;280(14):13424-32.

Bhave G, Zhu W, Wang H, Brasier DJ, Oxford GS, Gereau RWt. cAMP-dependent protein kinase regulates desensitization of the capsaicin receptor (VR1) by direct phosphorylation. Neuron 2002;35(4):721-31.

Mohapatra DP, Nau C. Desensitization of capsaicin-activated currents in the vanilloid receptor TRPV1 is decreased by the cyclic AMP-dependent protein kinase pathway. J Biol Chem 2003;278(50):50080-90.

Numazaki M, Tominaga T, Takeuchi K, Murayama N, Toyooka H, Tominaga M. Structural determinant of TRPV1 desensitization interacts with calmodulin. Proc Natl Acad Sci U S A 2003;100(13):8002-6.

Rosenbaum T, Gordon-Shaag A, Munari M, Gordon SE. Ca2+/calmodulin modulates TRPV1 activation by capsaicin. J Gen Physiol 2004;123(1):53-62.

Jung J, Shin JS, Lee SY, Hwang SW, Koo J, Cho H, et al. Phosphorylation of vanilloid receptor 1 by Ca2+/calmodulin-dependent kinase II regulates its vanilloid binding. J Biol Chem 2004;279(8):7048-54.

Remadevi R, Szallisi A. Adlea (ALGRX-4975), an injectable capsaicin (TRPV1 receptor agonist) formulation for longlasting pain relief. IDrugs 2008;11(2):120-32.

Szallasi A, Cruz F, Geppetti P. TRPV1: a therapeutic target for novel analgesic drugs? Trends Mol Med 2006;12(11):545-54.

Avelino A, Cruz F. TRPV1 (vanilloid receptor) in the urinary tract: expression, function and clinical applications. Naunyn Schmiedebergs Arch Pharmacol 2006;373(4):287-99.

Nolano M, Simone DA, Wendelschafer-Crabb G, Johnson T, Hazen E, Kennedy WR. Topical capsaicin in humans: parallel loss of epidermal nerve fibers and pain sensation. Pain 1999;81(1-2):135-45.

Di Marzo V, Blumberg PM, Szallasi A. Endovanilloid signaling in pain. Curr Opin Neurobiol 2002;12(4):372-79.

Bolcskei K, Helyes Z, Szabo A, Sandor K, Elekes K, Nemeth J, et al. Investigation of the role of TRPV1 receptors in acute and chronic nociceptive processes using gene-deficient mice. Pain 2005;117(3):368-76.

Wang X, Miyares RL, Ahern GP. Oleoylethanolamide excites vagal sensory neurones, induces visceral pain and reduces short-term food intake in mice via capsaicin receptor TRPV1. J Physiol 2005;564(Pt 2):541-47.

Christoph T, Bahrenberg G, De Vry J, Englberger W, Erdmann VA, Frech M, et al. Investigation of TRPV1 loss-of-function phenotypes in transgenic shRNA expressing and knockout mice. Mol Cell Neurosci 2008;37(3):579-89.

Klionsky L, Tamir R, Holzinger B, Bi X, Talvenheimo J, Kim H, et al. A polyclonal antibody to the prepore loop of transient receptor potential vanilloid type 1 blocks channel activation. J Pharmacol Exp Ther 2006;319(1):192-98.

Marincsak R, Toth BI, Czifra G, Szabo T, Kovacs L, Biro T. The analgesic drug, tramadol, acts as an agonist of the transient receptor potential vanilloid-1. Anesth Analg 2008;106(6):1890-6.

Mallet C, Barriere DA, Ermund A, Jonsson BA, Eschalier A, Zygmunt PM, et al. TRPV1 in brain is involved in acetaminophen-induced antinociception. PLoS One 2010;5(9).

Bertolini A, Ferrari A, Ottani A, Guerzoni S, Tacchi R, Leone S. Paracetamol: new vistas of an old drug. CNS Drug Rev 2006;12(3-4):250-75.

Verleye M, Gillardin JM. Contribution of transient receptor potential vanilloid subtype 1 to the analgesic and antihyperalgesic activity of nefopam in rodents. Pharmacology 2009;83(2):116-21.

Sui F, Zhang CB, Yang N, Li LF, Guo SY, Huo HR, et al. Anti-nociceptive mechanism of baicalin involved in intervention of TRPV1 in DRG neurons in vitro. J Ethnopharmacol 2010;129(3):361-66.

Sui F, Huo HR, Zhang CB, Yang N, Guo JY, Du XL, et al. Emodin down-regulates expression of TRPV1 mRNA and its function in DRG neurons in vitro. Am J Chin Med 2010;38(4):789-800.

Reynolds JEF. Martindale: the extra pharmacopoeia. Royal Pharmaceutical Society 1999;32nd edn.

Britain. BMARPSoG. British national formulary. BMA 2003; (No 45).

Campbell E, Bevan S, Dray A. Clinical applications of capsaicin and its analogues. In: JN W, editor. Capsaicin in the study of pain. London: Academic Press, 1993. 255-272.

Cantillon M, Hughes S, Moon A, Vause E, Sykes D. Safety, tolerability and efficacy of ALGRX 4975 in osteoarthritis of the knee. J Pain Off. J. Am. Pain Soc 2005;6(S39).

Diamond E, Richards P, Miller T. ALGRX 4975 reduces pain of intermetatarsal neuroma: preliminary results from a randomized, double-blind, placebo-controlled, phase II multicenter clinical trial. J Pain 2006;7(4):S41.

Richards P, Vasko G, IStasko I, Lacko M, Hewson G. (312/759): ALGRX 4975 reduces pain of acute lateral epicondylitis: Preliminary results from a randomized, double-blind, placebo-controlled, phase II multicenter clinical trial. J Pain 2006;7:S3.

Aasvang EK, Hansen JB, Malmstrom J, Asmussen T, Gennevois D, Struys MM, et al. The effect of wound instillation of a novel purified capsaicin formulation on postherniotomy pain: a double-blind, randomized, placebo-controlled study. Anesth Analg 2008;107(1):282-91.

Saper JR, Klapper J, Mathew NT, Rapoport A, Phillips SB, Bernstein JE. Intranasal civamide for the treatment of episodic cluster headaches. Arch Neurol 2002;59(6):990-04.

Diamond S, Freitag F, Phillips SB, Bernstein JE, Saper JR. Intranasal civamide for the acute treatment of migraine headache. Cephalalgia 2000;20(6):597-602.

ct2/results?term=civamide hwcg.

Backonja M, Wallace MS, Blonsky ER, Cutler BJ, Malan P, Jr., Rauck R, et al. NGX-4010, a high-concentration capsaicin patch, for the treatment of postherpetic neuralgia: a randomised, double-blind study. Lancet Neurol 2008;7(12):1106-12.

Backonja M. High-concentration capsaicin for the treatment of post-herpetic neuralgia and other types of peripheral neuropathic pain. European Journal of Pain Supplements 2010;4:170-74.

Noto C, Pappagallo M, Szallasi A. NGX-4010, a high-concentration capsaicin dermal patch for lasting relief of peripheral neuropathic pain. Curr Opin Investig Drugs 2009;10(7):702-10.

Simpson DM, Estanislao L, Brown SJ, Sampson J. An open-label pilot study of high-concentration capsaicin patch in painful HIV neuropathy. J Pain Symptom Manage 2008;35(3):299-306.

Webster LR, Malan TP, Tuchman MM, Mollen MD, Tobias JK, Vanhove GF. A multicenter, randomized, double-blind, controlled dose finding study of NGX-4010, a high-concentration capsaicin patch, for the treatment of postherpetic neuralgia. J Pain 2010;11(10):972-82.

Webster LR, Gazda SK, Medoff JR, Tobias J, Vanhove GF. NGX-4010, a High-Concentration Capsaicin Patch, in Painful Diabetic Neuropathy (PDN). In: American Academy of Pain Medicine (AAPM) 25th Annual Meeting; 2009; Honolulu, Hawaii; 2009.

Bevan S, Hothi S, Hughes G, James IF, Rang HP, Shah K, et al. Capsazepine: a competitive antagonist of the sensory neurone excitant capsaicin. Br J Pharmacol 1992;107(2):544-52.

Weil A, Moore SE, Waite NJ, Randall A, Gunthorpe MJ. Conservation of functional and pharmacological properties in the distantly related temperature sensors TRVP1 and TRPM8. Mol Pharmacol 2005;68(2):518-27.

Xing H, Chen M, Ling J, Tan W, Gu JG. TRPM8 mechanism of cold allodynia after chronic nerve injury. J Neurosci 2007;27(50):13680-90.

Holzer P. The pharmacological challenge to tame the transient receptor potential vanilloid-1 (TRPV1) nocisensor. Br J Pharmacol 2008;22:22.

Gavva NR, Tamir R, Klionsky L, Norman MH, Louis JC, Wild KD, et al. Proton activation does not alter antagonist interaction with the capsaicin-binding pocket of TRPV1. Mol Pharmacol 2005;68(6):1524-33.

Lehto SG, Tamir R, Deng H, Klionsky L, Kuang R, Le A, et al. Antihyperalgesic effects of (R,E)-N-(2-hydroxy-2,3-dihydro-1H-inden-4-yl)-3-(2-(piperidin-1-yl)-4-(trifluorom ethyl)phenyl)-acrylamide (AMG8562), a novel transient receptor potential vanilloid type 1 modulator that does not cause hyperthermia in rats. J Pharmacol Exp Ther 2008;326(1):218-29.

Seabrook GR, Sutton KG, Jarolimek W, Hollingworth GJ, Teague S, Webb J, et al. Functional properties of the high-affinity TRPV1 (VR1) vanilloid receptor antagonist (4-hydroxy-5-iodo-3-methoxyphenylacetate ester) iodo-resiniferatoxin. J Pharmacol Exp Ther 2002;303(3):1052-60.

Gavva NR, Klionsky L, Qu Y, Shi L, Tamir R, Edenson S, et al. Molecular determinants of vanilloid sensitivity in TRPV1. J Biol Chem 2004;279(19):20283-95.

Neelands TR, Jarvis MF, Han P, Faltynek CR, Surowy CS. Acidification of rat TRPV1 alters the kinetics of capsaicin responses. Mol Pain 2005;1:28.

Gunthorpe MJ, Rami HK, Jerman JC, Smart D, Gill CH, Soffin EM, et al. Identification and characterisation of SB-366791, a potent and selective vanilloid receptor (VR1/TRPV1) antagonist. Neuropharmacology 2004;46(1):133-49.

Behrendt HJ, Germann T, Gillen C, Hatt H, Jostock R. Characterization of the mouse cold-menthol receptor TRPM8 and vanilloid receptor type-1 VR1 using a fluorometric imaging plate reader (FLIPR) assay. Br J Pharmacol 2004;141(4):737-45.

Walker KM, Urban L, Medhurst SJ, Patel S, Panesar M, Fox AJ, et al. The VR1 antagonist capsazepine reverses mechanical hyperalgesia in models of inflammatory and neuropathic pain. J Pharmacol Exp Ther 2003;304(1):56-62.

Pomonis JD, Harrison JE, Mark L, Bristol DR, Valenzano KJ, Walker K. N-(4-Tertiarybutylphenyl)-4-(3-cholorphyridin-2-yl)tetrahydropyrazine -1(2H)-carbox-amide (BCTC), a novel, orally effective vanilloid receptor 1 antagonist with analgesic properties: II. in vivo characterization in rat models of inflammatory and neuropathic pain. J Pharmacol Exp Ther 2003;306(1):387-93.

Yamamoto W, Sugiura A, Nakazato-Imasato E, Kita Y. Characterization of primary sensory neurons mediating static and dynamic allodynia in rat chronic constriction injury model. J Pharm Pharmacol 2008;60(6):717-22.

Honore P, Wismer CT, Mikusa J, Zhu CZ, Zhong C, Gauvin DM, et al. A-425619 [1-isoquinolin-5-yl-3-(4-trifluoromethyl-benzyl)-urea], a novel transient receptor potential type V1 receptor antagonist, relieves pathophysiological pain associated with inflammation and tissue injury in rats. J Pharmacol Exp Ther 2005;314(1):410-21.

Swanson DM, Dubin AE, Shah C, Nasser N, Chang L, Dax SL, et al. Identification and biological evaluation of 4-(3-trifluoromethylpyridin-2-yl)piperazine-1-carboxylic acid (5-trifluoromethylpyridin-2-yl)amide, a high affinity TRPV1 (VR1) vanilloid receptor antagonist. J Med Chem 2005;48(6):1857-72.

Zhong C, Gauvin D, Mikusa J, Chandran P, Hernandez G, Lee L, et al. The novel and potent TRPV1 antagonist, A-784168, is a broad-spectrum analgesic in preclinical pain models. Washington, DC: Society for Neuroscience, 2005.

Trevisani M, Fruttarolo F, Pavani M, Campi B, Gatti R, De Siena G, et al. V377, a potent TRPV1 antagonist for pain management. European Opioid Conference (EOC) - European Neuropeptide Club (ENC) joint meeting. 2008.

Cui M, Honore P, Zhong C, Gauvin D, Mikusa J, Hernandez G, et al. TRPV1 receptors in the CNS play a key role in broad-spectrum analgesia of TRPV1 antagonists. J Neurosci 2006;26(37):9385-93.

Surowy CS, Neelands TR, Bianchi BR, McGaraughty S, El Kouhen R, Han P, et al. (R)-(5-tert-butyl-2,3-dihydro-1H-inden-1-yl)-3-(1H-indazol-4-yl)-urea (ABT-102) blocks polymodal activation of transient receptor potential vanilloid 1 receptors in vitro and heat-evoked firing of spinal dorsal horn neurons in vivo. J Pharmacol Exp Ther 2008;326(3):879-88.

Gomtsyan A, Bayburt EK, Schmidt RG, Surowy CS, Honore P, Marsh KC, et al. Identification of (R)-1-(5-tert-butyl-2,3-dihydro-1H-inden-1-yl)-3-(1H-indazol-4-yl)urea (ABT-102) as a potent TRPV1 antagonist for pain management. J Med Chem 2008;51(3):392-95.

Brown BS, Keddy R, Perner RJ, DiDomenico S, Koenig JR, Jinkerson TK, et al. Discovery of TRPV1 antagonist ABT-116. Bioorg Med Chem Lett. 2010 2010;20(11):3291-94.

Puttfarcken PS, Han P, Joshi SK, Neelands TR, Gauvin DM, Baker SJ, et al. A-995662 [(R)-8-(4-methyl-5-(4-(trifluoromethyl)phenyl)oxazol-2-ylamino)-1,2,3,4-tetrahydr onaphthalen-2-ol], a novel, selective TRPV1 receptor antagonist, reduces spinal release of glutamate and CGRP in a rat knee joint pain model. Pain 2010;150(2):319-26.

Wallace MS. Ziconotide: a new nonopioid intrathecal analgesic for the treatment of chronic pain. Expert Rev Neurother 2006;6(10):1423-28.

Menendez L, Juarez L, Garcia E, Garcia-Suarez O, Hidalgo A, Baamonde A. Analgesic effects of capsazepine and resiniferatoxin on bone cancer pain in mice. Neurosci Lett. 2006;393(1):70-3.

Brown DC, Iadarola MJ, Perkowski SZ, Erin H, Shofer F, Laszlo KJ, et al. Physiologic and antinociceptive effects of intrathecal resiniferatoxin in a canine bone cancer model. Anesthesiology 2005;103(5):1052-59.

Hori T. Capsaicin and central control of thermoregulation. Pharmacol Ther 1984;26(3):389-416.

Bannon A, Davis J, Zhu D, Norman M, Doherty E, Magal E, et al. Involvement of TRPV1 in the regulation of body temperature in rats and mice. In: Society for Neuroscience Annual Meeting Program; San Diego, CA; 2004.

Gavva NR, Bannon AW, Surapaneni S, Hovland Jr DN, Lehto SG, Gore A, et al. The Vanilloid Receptor TRPV1 Is Tonically Activated In Vivo and Involved in Body Temperature Regulation. J Neurosci 2007;27(13):3366 -74.

Romanovsky AA, Almeida MC, Garami A, Steiner AA, Norman MH, Morrison SF, et al. The transient receptor potential vanilloid-1 channel in thermoregulation: a thermosensor it is not. Pharmacol Rev 2009;61((3)):228-61.

Gavva NR. Body-temperature maintenance as the predominant function of the vanilloid receptor TRPV1. Trends Pharmacol Sci 2008;19:19.

Gavva NR, Treanor JJ, Garami A, Fang L, Surapaneni S, Akrami A, et al. Pharmacological blockade of the vanilloid receptor TRPV1 elicits marked hyperthermia in humans. Pain 2008;136(1-2):202-10.

Steiner AA, Turek VF, Almeida MC, Burmeister JJ, Oliveira DL, Roberts JL, et al. Nonthermal activation of transient receptor potential vanilloid-1 channels in abdominal viscera tonically inhibits autonomic cold-defense effectors. J Neurosci 2007;27(28):7459-68.

Gavva NR, Bannon AW, Hovland DN, Jr., Lehto SG, Klionsky L, Surapaneni S, et al. Repeated administration of vanilloid receptor TRPV1 antagonists attenuates hyperthermia elicited by TRPV1 blockade. J Pharmacol Exp Ther 2007;323(1):128-37.

Garcia-Martinez C, Humet M, Planells-Cases R, Gomis A, Caprini M, Viana F, et al. Attenuation of thermal nociception and hyperalgesia by VR1 blockers. Proc Natl Acad Sci USA 2002;99(4):2374-79.

Tang L, Chen Y, Chen Z, Blumberg PM, Kozikowski AP, Wang ZJ. Antinociceptive pharmacology of N-(4-chlorobenzyl)-N'-(4-hydroxy-3-iodo-5-methoxybenzyl) thiourea, a high-affinity competitive antagonist of the transient receptor potential vanilloid 1 receptor. J Pharmacol Exp Ther 2007;321(2):791-98.

Eid SR. To Feel or not to Feel - Targeting the Heat Sensor TRPV1 for Pain Treatment. In: Keystone meeting on Neurobiology of Pain and Analgesia. http://www.keystonesymposia.org; Santa Fe, New Mexico; 2009.

Chizh BA, Sang CN. Use of sensory methods for detecting target engagement in clinical trials of new analgesics. Neurotherapeutics 2009;6(4):749-54.

Eid SR. TRPV1 Antagonists: Are They Too Hot to Handle? In: 3rd annual Pain Therapeutics Summit in Summit. http://www.arrowheadpublishers. com/conferences/pain-therapeutics-2009/agenda/; 2009; Summit, New Jersey; 2009.

http://www.jt.com/investors/results/pharmaceuticals/pdf/P.L.20100729_E.pdf

http://www.qutenza.com/.

Chapter II

Allodynia and neuronal plasticity

*Ricardo A Cruciani, MD, PhD[*1,2,3], Charles B Stacy[4], MD, Seth A Resnick[1,5,6], MD and Helena Knotkova, PhD[1,2]*

[1]Institute for Non-invasive Brain Stimulation, Research Division,
Department of Pain Medicine and Palliative Care,
Beth Israel Medical Center, New York, New York, US
[2]Department of Neurology, Albert Einstein College of Medicine,
Bronx, New York, US
[3]Department of Anesthesiology, Albert Einstein College of Medicine,
Bronx, New York, US
[4]Department of Neurology, Mount Sinai Medical Center, and
[5]Continuum Cancer Centers of New York, New York, US
[6] Department of Psychiatry, Albert Einstein College of Medicine,
Bronx, New York, US

Abstract

Neuropathic pain is typically acccompanied by a constelation of signs and symptoms that gives to this condition a very distinct presentation.

---

[*] Correspondence: Ricardo A Cruciani, MD, PhD, Institute for Non-invasive Brain Stimulation, Research Division, Department of Pain Medicine and Palliative Care, Beth Israel Medical Center, 350 E 17th Street, Baird Hall, 12th fl., New York, NY, 10003, United States. E-mail: RCrucian@chpnet.org

Allodynia – pain sensation induced by non-noxious stimuli, along with hyperalgesia – an exaggerated response to noxious stimuli, are common findings in neuropathic pain, and are frequently accompanied by dysesthesias, paresthesias, after-sensations, and less frequently by changes in coloration and temperature of the affected area. Both hyperalgesia and allodynia are of special interest becuase they seem to be sensory expressions of very complex underlying phenomena. This article discusses neural mechanisms in the development and maintenance of allodynia, and the role of peripheral- and central sensitization in sensory disturbances present in neuropathic pain.

Introduction

Tissue or nerve injury, inflamation and infections, can lead to pain that outlasts the duration of the insult and may be accompanied by an abnormal sensory response. This type of pain is called neuropathic in counterposition to nociceptive that is a normal selfprotective response to a noxious stimuli (1). Neuropathic pain is typically acccompanied by a constelation of signs and symptoms than when all present, gives to this condition a very distinct presentation. In ocassions only subtle changes are evident making the diagnosis challenging. Allodynia, along with hyperalgesia, are common findings in this abnormal response to a sensory stimuli, and are frequently accompanied by dysesthesias, paresthesias, after-sensations, and less frequently by changes in coloration and temperature of the affected area (see table 1).

Both hyperalgesia and allodynia are of special interest becuase they seem to be sensory expressions of very complex underlying phenomena. Hyperalgesia is an exaggerated painful response to painful stimuli while allodynia is an abnormal perception of pain to nonpainful stimuli. Allodynia can be clasified into mechanical or thermal depending on the stimulus that provoques it. In addtion, mechanical allodynia can be subdivided into static (pain provoqued by gentle pressure on the skin), and dynamic (pain provoked by light brushing)(2). Both sensations, light pressure and touch, are normally transmitted by a different types of fibers (Aβ fibers), that are myelinated and have a lower treshold to stimualtion than those transmitting pain signals (C fibers, non myelinated). In order for the Aβ fibers, that normally transmit mechanical information, to trasnmit pain information, they either have to change their conductive and receptive properties at the level of the peripheral nervous system, or change the intrepretation of the sensory information at the level of the central nervous system. The other type of allodynia, thermal, can be clasified into heat and cold.

Table 1. Terms that are commonly utilized in neuropathic pain and central sensitization

Nociceptive pain	Normal painful sensation due to noxious stimuli. Pain is triggered by peripheral stimuli and is proportional to its intensity and duration.
Neuropathic pain	Abnormal response to noxious stimuli.
Noxiuos stimuli	Stimuli that activates nociceptors (with or without tissue injury).
Nociceptors	Naked terminals that are activated by noxious stimuli. When activated they produce a sensation of pain. They are localized in most structures including nerves (nervo nervorum).
Allodynia	Painful sensation to a non-painful stimulation: mechanical, thermal. When present, suggestive of central sensitization.
Hyperalgesia	Exaggerated painful response to painful stimuli.
Hyperesthesia	Increased sensation to a stimuli.
Primary hyperalgesia	Increased painful sensation at the level of the lesion. Caused by decreased threshold of nociceptors and increased response.
Secondary hyperalgesia	Increased painful response distant to the area of the lesion.
Hyperpathia	Exaggerated pain reaction caused by a repetitive non-painful stimulation.
Dysesthesias	An unpleasant sensory sensation evoked by a stimuli that normally would cause a different sensory response.
Paresthesias	Sensory sensation in the absence of stimuli.
Central sensitization	Activity dependent synaptic plasticity at any level of the CNS. Studied in detail in the spinal cord.
Windup	Increase in response at the level of the post horn of the spinal cord, due to repeated low frequency stimulation of c fibers.
Peripheral sensitization	Increased response to noxious stimuli at the level of the affected area. Decreased threshold (more to heat stimuli).

Cold allodynia can present differently upon the injury that casues it. In patients with neuropathic pain, cold allodynia is usually present along with other signs of central excitability like hyperalgesia, while in patients with permanent injury induced by prolonged exposure to low temperature it seems to be due to peripheral mechanisms only.

When the changes responsible for the modification of the noxious response are localized in the periphery, we call that phenomenon peripheral sensitization, a change in properties that succesfully explains an exaggerated response to the same repetitive painful stimulation, to increased pain in the area of inflamattion, but does not explain some other phenomena like allodynia. The mechanisms underlying this change in the sensory response that leads to peripheral sensitization includes:

1. release of endogenous algogenic chemicals including serotonin, prostaglandins, substance P, K+, protons and histamine, all causing directly or indirectly increaed responsivness of the skin;
2. lowering the membrane thresholds; 3) long-lasting changes in neurotransmitter levels localized to the site of injury. This phenomenon was studied in normal volunteers by injection of capsaicin and the development of concetric areas of hperalgesia and allodynia has been observed (see figure 1).

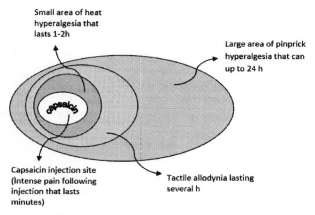

Figure 1. Cutaneous hyperalgesia induced by capsaicin injection. Effect of intradermal administration of capsaicin. Shortly after the injection of capsaicin, pain in the area of the injection develops. The pain is intense and lasts for about an hour. This area is surrounded by a small region of hyperalgesia, that is folowed by an area of allodynia and outermost another area of hyperalgesia. The outermost area cannot be explained by changes in the preriphery and represents central sensitization.

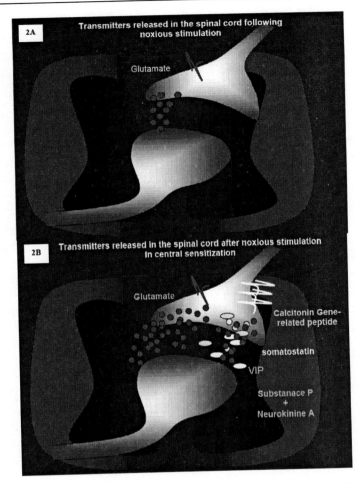

Figure 2. Representation of a glutaminergic synapsis at the level of the lamina II where the first neuron synapses with the projection neuron. 2A. Following noxious stimuli in the peripjhery, the neurotransmitter glutamate is released, producing activation of NMDA receptors at the level of the postsynapsis convening noxious stimuli to the CNS by synapsing with a third neuron that is localized in the thalamus. The pathways ends in the sensory are located in the precentral sulcus. 2B. Repetitive stimulation of the afferent fibers causes exagerated response of the glutaminergic neuron causing additional release of glutamate. This in terms is accompanied or followed by other peptides that contribute to a robust response. This mechanism is believed to participate also in the recruitment of fibers that normally do not transmit noxious information (e.g. A beta fibers that transmit mechanical information). In addition to glutamate (the major neurotrnamitter at this level), in states of central sensitization substance P, neurokinin A, VIP, calcitonin gene related peptide, and somatostatin may contribute to the response.

Other changes also occur, such as an expression of sodium channels at the lesion site that cause an increase in spontaneous activity and ectopic firing in the stump of the injured nerves that then expands to intact structures lowering the nociceptor threshold, increasing their response to suprathreshold stimuli. In inflammatory pain like arthritis, the mechanism of primary sensitization is somehow different with a preponderant role for prostaglandines.

Central sensitization, on the other hand, refers to an increase in the functional status of neurons and circuits in nociceptive pathways throughout the central nervous system caused by increases in membrane excitability, synaptic efficacy, or reduced inhibition, and may recruit pathways not otherwise activated by such inputs (see figure 2)(1,2).

Recently the complexity of the phenomenon has become appreciated, and includes activity-dependent synaptic plasticity; the long term potentiation, changes in microglia, astrocytes, gap junctions, membrane excitability and gene transcription all can contribute to the maintenance of central sensitization (3-12).

Long term potentiation (LTP) in central sensitization

Enhancement of transmission at the level of the excitatory synapses occurs through several mechanisms including long-term potentiation. The prototypical form of long-term potentiation is the one described in the hippocampus and is induced by repeated trains of high frequency stimuli, causing post-synaptic AMPA activation by glutamate, opening of sodium ion channels, and allowing summation of EPSPs. EPSPs sumation eventually produces sufficient depolarization that unblocks NMDA receptors that is followed by calcium influx in the presence of glutamate. This in turn activates protein kinase C, calcium/calmodulin dependent protein kinase II, and to a lesser extent mitogen-activated protein kinase (MAPK), and protein kinase A. This early phase of long-term potentiation is maintained by activation of Protein Kinase M zeta, which does not depend on continued calcium influx. These activated kinases phosphorylate AMPA receptors, increasing their activity, while promoting the insertion of additional AMPA receptors into the post synaptic membrane. The late phase of long-term potentiation involves gene transcription and protein synthesis in the post synaptic cells, which are consequences of persistent activation of MAPK, particularly the extracellular signal related kinase (ERK) subfamily, coincident with PKA activation and calcium influx(1). Ultimately, the maintenance of long-term potentiation may depend on the constitutively active PKM zeta, the induction of pre-synaptic protein synthesis, and dendritically local post-synaptic protein synthesis. This mechanism of homosynaptic potentiation is not likely to be the only means of central sensitization, as it depends on high frequency nociceptive firing. Heterosynaptic potentiation, illustrated by the expansion of receptor fields and the activation of nociceptive pathways by normally non-noxious stimuli that leads in the activation of nociceptive pathways by normally non- innocuous stimuli, is presumably the more common situation, as it can be evoked by less intense inputs. C fiber activation readily induces central sensitization even at low firing rates though the mediation of NMDA receptors. Summation of slow synaptic potentials unblocks the NMDA channel by magnesium, and also enhances NMDA function through G protein coupled receptors and receptor tyrosine kinases and by MAPK phosphorylation.In addition, AMPA receptors which lack the edited form of Glu R2 subunits permit calcium entry, thus triggering the mechanisms for long-term synaptic facilitation (2).

Homosynaptic changes will contribute with peripheral sensitization to primary hyperalgesia (13,14) whereas heterosynaptic facilitation alone is responsible for secondary hyperalgesia and allodynia. Interestingly, heterosynaptic facilitation has not been described in the hipoccampus. The mediators of heterosynaptic facilitation involve most likely activated mGluRs and NO. mGluRs are coupled to the Ca channels of the endoplasmic reticulum and play an important role in central sensitization (15). Consequently, the release of intracellular Ca in spinal cord neurons on mGluR activation may participate in spreading facilitation from conditioned synapses to neighboring test synapses. NO is also a major effectors of spinal cord neuronal plasticity (16,17)) and diffuses rapidly from the site of its production to produce multiple effects at a distance via its downstream signaling pathways, and in this way may contribute to the heterosynaptic facilitation characteristic of central sensitization. It is certainly likely that these and other ''spreading'' signals cooperate to produce the widespread synaptic facilitation so characteristic to central sensitization. Scaffolding proteins play a major role in the addressing of specific kinases to the synapse and represent another potential mechanism for widespread synaptic facilitation. A recent study has shown that in the hippocampus, CaMKII activation is restricted to the synaptic button of a conditioned synapse, thus only allowing homosynaptic facilitation at that specific site (18). It is likely in the dorsal horn that CaMKII activation

Role of the glia in central sensitization

Traditional thinking has taught for years that only neurons and neural circuits mediated pain, and glial cells served only as a structural support for neurons. However, the current thinking is that glial cells are active and that they interact with neurons, regulate their milieu and have the ability to respond to environmental changes. Rather than neurons regulating glial activity or vise versa, there is an ongoing dialogue between the two. Indeed, glial cells express various types of neurotransmitter receptors that enable them to respond to neural signals and also produce numerous mediators including proinflammatory cytokines and growth factors that regulate neuronal activity. The glial cell population in the CNS is formed by three types of cells: microglia, astrocytes and oligodendrocytes. The microglial cells are derived from bone marrow precursors and it is now accepted that they actively participate in the regulation of brain function (19). Recently, evidence has accumulated that supports a role of spinal microglia in the development of neuropathic pain. Nerve injury induces the expression of microglial markers (e.g. CD11b, TLR4 and CD14) (20) and microgial activation including upregulation of chemokine receptor CX3CR1 and ATP receptor P2X4 receptors that results in astrocyte activation (21). Deletion or blockade of these receptors results in decreased neuropathic pain (22-25). There is additional evidence that demonstrate an involvement of the microglia in the pain response including non-specific microglial inhibition with minocycline that prevents the pain development (26-28) intrathecal injection of ATP-activated microglia that induces mechanical allodynia through the production of microglial BDNF (29,30) and reversal of hypersensititiv by blockade of p38 mitogen-activated protein kinase (MAPK) that can occur in several chronic pain conditions (Table 1) (31-35). A recent study shows that a nerve-injury induced cleavage of the chemokine fractalkine results in activation of p38 in spinal microglia via CX3CR1 receptors (36).

Astrocytes are closely associated to neurons and blood vessels as suggested by its parallel metabolic activity with that in neurons. The role of astrocites in the genesis and regulation of chronic pain was initially made evident by manipulating astrocytic metabolism (37,38) and more recently by the observation that proinflammatory cytokines such as interleukin 1b (IL-1b),

IL-6 and tumor necrosis factor a (TNF-a) are produced in glial cells and upregulated in the spinal cord in chronic pain conditions. Furthermore, functional inhibition of these cytokines can attenuate persistent pain and enhance opioid analgesia (39-42). In addition allodynia can be reversed through the inhibition of glial function by spinal delivery of specific glial inhibitors (e.g. propentofylline)(43). Propentofylline, an atypical methylxantine attenuates a nerve injury-induced astrocytic and microglial activation (44) and also suppresses the expression of tumor necrosis factor-α and interleukin (IL)-1β, IL-6 (pro-inflammatory cytokines)(45).

Role of sodium channels

Changes in the properties of the voltage sensitive sodium channels has been described both in the DRG neurons and the sensory nerve fibers as well. In neuromas, nerve structures that forms in the proximal end of a transected nerve as part of the healing process, grouping and changes of the sodium channel properties has also been described. The sodium channels seem to play a role in both the development of peripheral and central sensitization. The identification of a variety of voltage sensitive sodium channels, Na_v 1.7, that is present in sensory neurons dorsal root ganglia, sympathetic neurons, Schwann cells, and neuroendocrine cells, but not in the heart of the CNS, has developed special interest in this field. It was hypothesized that the development of selective channel blockers for the variant of voltage gated sodium channel Na_v 1.7 would represent an unprecedented opportunity to block responses to noxious stimuli without causing significant side effects (46). However, in chronic pain states like neuropathic pain, there are significant changes in this receptor type making this strategy less promising than originally anticipated. In neuropathic pain models, the sodium channels undergo significant changes: 1) a "regression" to early forms of the receptor that is less stable, with a lower threshold and more excitable; 2) an appearance of other variants that are also present in cardiac and CNS tissue making them susceptible to side effects when blocked (Na_v 1.8 and Na_v 1.9). These changes not only occur in the injured nerve fibers but also occur in "surviving" uninjured fibers (Figure 3 and 4).

Other channels receiving attention at this time for the potential role in allodynia and hyperalgesia are the calcium and potassium channels.

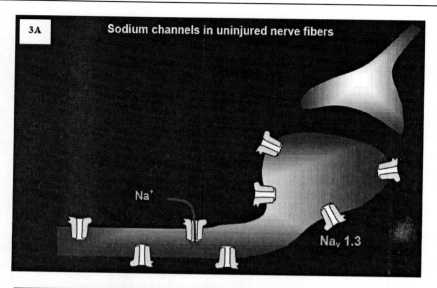

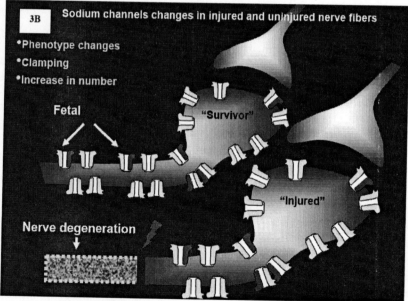

Figure 3. Representation of a sensory fiber and the role of the sodium channels in the nerve transmission. 3A. In a normal fiber the voltage sensitive sodium channels participate in the propagation of the action potentials that are elicited by noxius stimuli. 3B. After a nerve injury the number of sodium channels increase, the channels clamp, and other fenotypes that are not present in the adult appear. Interestingly changes are also observed in the surviving fibers.

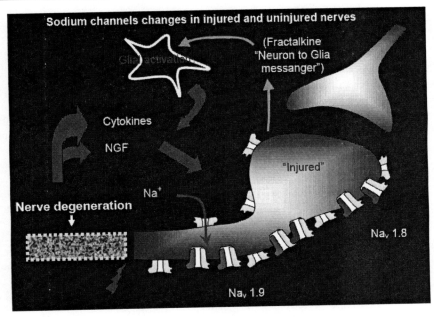

Figure 4. "Conversation" between neurons and the surounding glia. Subsequent to a nerve injury (e.g. a disc pressing on a root), cytokines and neural growth factors (NGF) are released. An additional stimulation comes from the intact portion of the neuron that produces fractalkin (a neural glial messenger). The glia produces cytokines and NGF that acts on the affected neuron and the surrounding "survivors" contributing to the changes in sodium channels and other modulators.

Conclusions

Neuropathic pain, an abnormal response to a sensory stimulus, can be very difficult to treat due to the complex underlying mechanism. Two phenomena showed to be critical to its complexity: peripheral and central sensitization. The ability of the CNS and peripheral nervous system to change sensitivity and recruit circuitries with other functions than pain transmission to elicit painful responses to noxious and non-noxious stimuli underscores the plasticity of the pain system.

References

[1] Latremoliere A and Woolf CJ. Central Sensitization: A generator of pain hypersensitivity by central neural plasticity. J Pain 2009;10(9):895-926.

[2] Woolf CJ. Central sensitization: Implications for the diagnosis and treatment of pain. Pain 2010 Oct 18. [Epub ahead of print]

[3] 3.Chacur M, Lambertz D, Hoheisel U, Mense S. Role of spinal microglia in myositis-induced central sensitisation: An immunohistochemical and behavioural study in rats. Eur J Pain 2009;13:915–23.

[4] Chang YW and Waxman SG. Minocycline attenuates mechanical allodynia and central sensitization following peripheral second-degree burn injury. J Pain 2010; doi:10.1016/j.jpain.2010.02.010.

[5] Chiang CY, Li Z, Dostrovsky JO, Sessle BJ. Central sensitization in medullary dorsal horn involves gap junctions and hemichannels. Neuroreport 2010;21:233–7.

[6] Chiechio S, Zammataro M, Morales ME, Busceti CL, Drago F. Gereau RWT, Copani A, Nicoletti F. Epigenetic modulation of mGlu2 receptors by histone deacetylase inhibitors in the treatment of inflammatory pain. Mol Pharmacol 2009;75:1014–20.

[7] Gao YJ, Zhang L, Samad OA, Suter MR, Yasuhiko K, Xu ZZ, Park JY, Lind AL, Ma Q, Ji RR. JNK-induced MCP-1 production in spinal cord astrocytes contributes to central sensitization and neuropathic pain. J Neurosci 2009;29:4096–108.

[8] Hathway GJ, Vega-Avelaira D, Moss A, Ingram R, Fitzgerald M. Brief, low frequency stimulation of rat peripheral C-fibres evokes prolonged microglialinduced central sensitization in adults but not in neonates. Pain 2009;144:110–8.

[9] Rivera-Arconada I and Lopez-Garcia JA. Changes in membrane excitability and potassium currents in sensitized dorsal horn neurons of mice pups. J Neurosci 2010;30:5376–83.

[10] Samad TA, Moore KA, Sapirstein A, Billet S, Allchorne A, Poole S, Bonventre JV, Woolf CJ. Interleukin-1beta-mediated induction of Cox-2 in the CNS contributes to inflammatory pain hypersensitivity. Nature 2001;410:471–5.

[11] Seybold VS. The role of peptides in central sensitization. Handb Exp Pharmacol 2009;194:451–91.

[12] Torres TM and Roman RD. Risk of transmission of human immunodeficiency virus type 1 after accidents with needles from drug addicts, occurred in the community. Rev Clin Esp 1991;189:95–6.

[13] Ikeda H, Stark J, Fischer H, Wagner M, Drdla R, Jager T, Sandkuhler J: Synaptic amplifier of inflammatory pain in the spinal dorsal horn. Science 2006;312:1659-62.

[14] Sandkuhler J: Understanding LTP in pain pathways. Mol Pain 2007;3:9.

[15] Adwanikar H, Karim F, Gereau RW: Inflammation persistently enhances nocifensive behaviors mediated by spinal group I mGluRs through sustained ERK activation. Pain 2004;111:125-35.

[16] Moreno-Lopez B and Gonzalez-Forero D: Nitric oxide and synaptic dynamics in the adult brain: Physiopathological aspects. Rev Neurosci 2006;17:309-57.

[17] Susswein AJ, Katzoff A, Miller N, Hurwitz I: Nitric oxide and memory. Neuroscientist 2004;10:153-62.

Allodynia and neuronal plasticity 45

[18] Lee SJ, Escobedo-Lozoya Y, Szatmari EM, Yasuda R: Activation of CaMKII in single dendritic spines during long-term potentiation. Nature 458:299-304, 2009.

[19] Nimmerjahn A, Kirchhoff F, Helmchen F. Resting microglial cells are highly dynamic surveillants of brain parenchyma in vivo. Science 2005;308:1314–18.

[20] DeLeo JA, Tanga FY, Tawfik VL. Neuroimmune activation and neuroinflammation in chronic pain and opioid tolerance/hyperalgesia. Neuroscientist 2004;10:40–52.

[21] Aldskogius H and Kozlova EN. Central neuron-glial and glialglial interactions following axon injury. Progress in Neurobology 1998;55:1–26.

[22] Tsuda M, Shigemoto-Mogami Y, Koizumi S, Mizokoshi A, Kohsaka S, Salter MW. P2X4 receptors induced in spinal microglia gate tactile allodynia after nerve injury. Nature 2004;424: 778–83.

[23] Milligan ED, Zapata V, Chacur M, Schoeniger D, Biedenkapp J, O'Connor KA, Verge G.M. Evidence that exogenous and endogenous fractalkine can induce spinal nociceptive facilitation in rats. Eur J Neurosci 2004;20:2294–2302.

[24] Verge GM, Milligan ED, Maier SF, Watkins LR, Naeve GS, Foster AC. Fractalkine (CX3CL1) and fractalkine receptor (CX3CR1) distribution in spinal cord and dorsal root ganglia under basal and neuropathic pain conditions. Eur J Neurosci 2004;20:1150–60.

[25] Zhuang ZY, Kawasaki Y, Tan PH, Wen YR, Huang J, Ji RR. Role of the CX3CR1/p38 MAPK pathway in spinal microglia for the development of neuropathic pain following nerve injuryinduced cleavage of fractalkine. Brain Behav Immunity 2006.

[26] Raghavendra V, Tanga F, DeLeo JA. Inhibition of microglial activation attenuates the development but not existing hypersensitivity in a rat model of neuropathy. J Pharmacol Exp Therapeutics 2003;306:624–30.

[27] Ledeboer A, Sloane EM, Milligan ED, Frank MG, Mahony JH, Maier SF. Minocycline attenuates mechanical allodynia and proinflammatory cytokine expression in rat models of pain facilitation. Pain 2005;115:71–83.

[28] Hua XY, Svensson CI, Matsui T, Fitzsimmons B, Yaksh TL, Webb M. Intrathecal minocycline attenuates peripheral inflammation-induced hyperalgesia by inhibiting p38 MAPK in spinal microglia. Eur J Neurosci 2005;22:2431–40.

[29] Tsuda M, Shigemoto-Mogami Y, Koizumi S, Mizokoshi A, Kohsaka S, Salter MW. P2X4 receptors induced in spinal microglia gate tactile allodynia after nerve injury. Nature 2003;424:778–83.

[30] Coull JA, Beggs S, Boudreau D, Boivin D, Tsuda M, Inoue K. BDNF from microglia causes the shift in neuronal anion gradient underlying neuropathic pain. Nature 2005;438:1017–21.

[31] Jin SX, Zhuang ZY, Woolf CJ, Ji RR. P38 mitogenactivated protein kinase is activated after a spinal nerve ligation in spinal cord microglia and dorsal root ganglion neurons and contributes to the generation of neuropathic pain. J Neurosci 2003;23:4017–22.

[32] Schafers M, Svensson CI, Sommer C, Sorkin LS. Tumor necrosis factor-alpha induces mechanical allodynia after spinal nerve ligation by activation of p38 MAPK in primary sensory neurons. J Neurosci 2003;23:2517–21.

[33] Tsuda M, Mizokoshi A, Shigemoto-Mogami Y, Koizumi S, Inoue K. Activation of p38 mitogen-activated protein kinase in spinal hyperactive microglia contributes to pain hypersensitivity following peripheral nerve injury. Glia 2004;45:89–95.

[34] Boyle DL, Jones TL, Hammaker D, Svensson CI, Rosengren S, Albani S. Regulation of Peripheral Inflammation by Spinal p38 MAP Kinase in Rats. PLoS Med 2006;3:e338.

[35] Hains BC and Waxman SG. Activated microglia contribute to the maintenance of chronic pain after spinal cord injury. J Neurosci 2006;26:4308–17.

[36] Haydon PG and Carmignoto G. Astrocyte control of synaptic transmission and neurovascular coupling. Physiol Rev 2006;86:1009–31.

[37] Meller ST, Dykstra C, Grzybycki D, Murphy S, Gebhart GF. The possible role of glia in nociceptive processing and hyperalgesia in the spinal cord of the rat. Neuropharmacol 1994;33:1471–8.

[38] Watkins LR, Martin D, Ulrich P, Tracey KJ, Maier SF. Evidence for the involvement of spinal cord glia in subcutaneous formalin induced hyperalgesia in the rat. Pain 1997;71:225–35.

[39] Sweitzer S, Martin D, DeLeo JA. Intrathecal interleukin-1 receptor antagonist in combination with soluble tumor necrosis factor receptor exhibits an anti-allodynic action in a rat model of neuropathic pain. Neuroscience 2001;103:529–39.

[40] Watkins LR, Milligan ED, Maier SF. Glial activation: a driving force for pathological pain. Trends Neurosci 2001;24:450–55.

[41] Milligan ED, Twining C, Chacur M, Biedenkapp J, O'Connor K, Poole S. Spinal glia and proinflammatory cytokines mediate mirror-image neuropathic pain in rats. J Neurosci 2003;23:1026–40.

[42] Watkins LR, Hutchinson MR, Johnston IN, Maier SF. Glia: novel counter-regulators of opioid analgesia. Trends Neurosci 2005;28:661–69.

[43] Milligan ED and Watkins LR. Pathological and protective roles of glia in chronic pain. Nat. Rev. Neuroscience 2009;10:23–36.

[44] Sweitzer SM, Schubert P, DeLeo JA. Propentofylline, a glial modulating agent, exhibits antiallodynic properties in a rat model of neuropathic pain. J Pharmacol Exp Ther 2001;297: 1210–7.

[45] Raghavendra V, Tanga F, Rutkowski MD, DeLeo JA. Antihyperalgesic and morphine-sparing actions of propentofylline following peripheral nerve injury in rats: mechanistic implications of spinal glia and proinflammatory cytokines. Pain 2003;104:655–64.

[46] Cox JJ, Reiman F, Nichola AK, Thornton G, Roberts E, Springell K, Karbani G, Jafri H. An *SCN9A* channelopathy causes congenital inability to experience pain. Nature 2006;444:894-98.

Chapter III

Spinal cord neural plasticity in chronic pain and its clinical implication

Jacqueline R Dauch, BS and Hsinlin T Cheng, MD, PhD[*]
University of Michigan, Department of Neurology,
Ann Arbor, Michigan, US

Abstract

Chronic pain is a common medical condition that causes significant physical and psychological disabilities to the general population. Although there is a high prevalence of chronic pain, effective treatments are still in urgent need to treat the condition. Fortunately, researchers have shed light on the molecular mechanism of painful chronic conditions for both inflammatory and neuropathic pain through recent animal studies. Through these studies, researchers have discovered that the spinal cord is an important relay center to integrate peripheral painful inputs and propagate signals to the brain. In painful conditions, peripheral nociceptors transmit afferent painful signals to the spinal cord dorsal horn (SCDH) by releasing neurotransmitters from presynaptic terminals. These neurotransmitters cross the synapse and activate the corresponding

---

[*] Correspondence: Hsinlin T Cheng MD, PhD, University of Michigan, Department of Neurology, 109 Zina Pitcher Place, 5015 BSRB, Ann Arbor, MI 48109, United States. E-mail: chengt@umich.edu

receptors on the postsynaptic terminals of neurons and glial cells in the SCDH. These events induce multiple inflammatory and neuropathic processes in the SCDH, as well as trigger modification and plasticity of local neural circuits. In addition, the activation of glial cells, including astrocytes and microglia in SCDH, contribute to the persistence of increased nociception through the enhancement of local actions of cytokines and chemokines. As a result of such molecular modifications, painful signals are often amplified and prolonged, a phenomenon known as central sensitization. In this review, the molecular events associated with central sensitization and their clinical implications are discussed.

Introduction

Pain is defined as "an unpleasant sensory and emotional experience associated with actual or potential tissue damage, or described in terms of such damage" by the international association for the study of pain (www.iasp-pain.org). Nociception, or pain perception, is a protective mechanism for preventing potential damage to an organism. It is essential for an organism to detect harmful stimuli and to respond adequately for survival. This sensory function is mediated by transmission of electrical and chemical signals through the neural axis to the brain. Such signals originate from peripheral nerve endings, pass through the spinal cord (SC), relay in the thalamus, and eventually reach the sensory cortex. Along this nociception pathway, the SC is an important entry site due to the fact that it is the location of the integration of primary sensory inputs and further propagation to the central nervous system.

Noxious signals, which are originally generated from peripheral sensory afferents in the SC, travel through synapses and then are transmitted to secondary sensory neurons in superficial layers of the SC dorsal horn (SCDH). Such neurons then transmit the noxious signal through ascending pathways to higher levels of the nervous system. Multiple pre- and postsynaptic inputs affect synapses between primary sensory inputs and sensory neurons in the SCDH. This network involves signals from local SC interneurons and other sensory neurons from deeper layers of the SCDH. In addition, there are descending pathways from the brain that serve as modulators for adjusting output signals of the SCDH projection neurons. Integration of these complex mechanisms contributes to normal nociception. Additionally, there are glial cells in the nervous system that contribute to nociception. They regulate neural activity along the neurons and nerve tracts that transmit pain signals. Normal nociceptive function is dependent on the balanced actions of each individual system.

In states of chronic inflammatory or neuropathic pain, normal nociceptive function may become altered in order to induce abnormal sensory phenomena such as allodynia and hyperalgesia. Allodynia describes an increased nociception to normally innocuous stimuli (eg. light touch), and hyperalgesia defines an excessive painful response to a painful stimulus (eg. pinprick). Abnormal nociception involves plasticity by altering multiple neuro-transmitters and intracellular signaling events in the SCDH and is termed central sensitization (1). Alterations in the production and secretion of neurotransmitters, neuropeptides, cytokines, chemokines, and growth factors, change the expression or activity of receptors for secreted ligands. Frank changes in physical interactions between cells, such as axonal sprouting, contribute to the development of central sensitization. This review outlines current knowledge on the molecular and cellular events involved in the process of central sensitization within the SC, as well as prospects for targeting these processes in the clinical treatment of chronic pain.

Normal pain physiology

Peripheral nerves for nociception

In response to painful stimuli, action potentials are transmitted along sensory fibers to cell bodies of corresponding primary sensory neurons in the dorsal root ganglia (DRG). The main peripheral nerve fibers for nociception are made up of Aδ and C fibers. These primary sensory afferent fibers carry painful signals from peripheral mechanical, thermal, and chemical stimuli. After converging afferent noxious signals from their peripheral processes, DRG neurons translate these electric pain signals and convert them into chemical signals by secreting neurotransmitters and neuropeptides into the SCDH. In general, peripheral afferent pain fibers can be divided into peptidergic and nonpeptidergic fibers, depending on their ability to express neuropeptides.

Glutamate is the primary neurotransmitter expressed by nonpeptidergic fibers. These fibers are dependent on glial cell-derived neurotrophic factor (GDNF) during embryonic development. In contrast, peptidergic fibers are nerve growth factor (NGF)-dependent and secrete both glutamate and neuropeptides, including substance P (SP) and calcitonin gene-related peptide (CGRP). After painful stimuli, these neurotransmitters and neuropeptides are released from presynaptic terminals in the superficial layers of the SCDH, diffuse across synaptic clefts, and bind to postsynaptic receptors on secondary sensory neurons (see Figure 1).

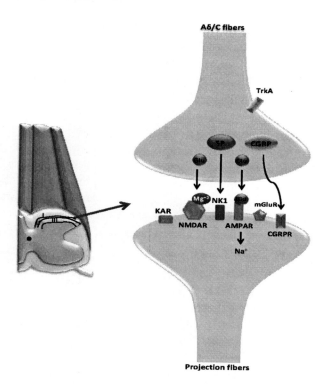

Figure 1. Normal nociceptive pathways in SCDH. In the superficial laminae, incoming Trk A-positive Aδ and C fibers carry nociceptive signals from peripheral nerves. These presynaptic terminals use glutamate, SP, or CGRP as nociceptive mediators. After painful stimulation, the mediators are released into synaptic clefts and interact with postsynaptic corresponding receptors. Most glutamate actions are mediated by AMPA receptor. In contrast, the NMDA receptor is blocked by physiological levels of Mg^{+2}.

Spinal circuits for pain processing

The second location for nociception transmission is the SCDH. Specific actions take place in certain levels of the SCDH which can be divided into several layers labeled "laminae" based on to their cellular structures according to Rexed (2). Most primary nociceptive fibers synapse with secondary neurons and interneurons in laminae I and II. Nearly all of these secondary nociceptive neurons and interneurons express the NK1 receptor and the receptor for SP. As a result, such neurons respond to the neurotransmitters and neuropeptides that are secreted from the nerve endings of DRG neurons (3, 4). In addition, NK1-positive neurons in the deeper layers of the SCDH also synapse with peptidergic sensory fibers in laminae I (3, 4). At another level, NK1-negative sensory neurons in laminae II of the SCDH receive input signals from nonpeptidergic afferent fibers. Dendrites from these NK1-negative neurons interact with NK1-positive neurons located in laminae I. In order to inhibit excessive nociceptive signals, sensory neurons in laminae I and II serve as local modulators and interact with GABAergic and glycinergic interneurons in laminae II and III (see figure 2) (5,6).

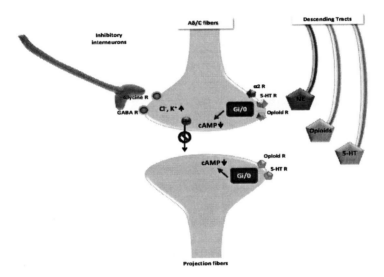

Figure 2. Local inhibitory circuits and descending pathways modulate nociception in SCDH. The inhibitory interneurons in the superficial layers of SCDH interact with presynaptic terminals by secreting GABA and glycine. These inhibitory neurotransmitters bind to their corresponding receptors on the presynaptic terminals and open the K^+ and Cl^- channels. As a result, the presynaptic membrane is hyperpolarized, resulting in decreased glutamate release and postsynaptic action potentials. The descending inhibitory pathways provide norepinephrine (NE), serotonin (5-HT), and endogenous opioids in SCDH. They interact with their corresponding pre and post-synaptic receptors to decrease membranous action potentials by $G_i/0$ protein and cAMP mediated mechanisms.

The net actions from all these neural circuits determine the ultimate merging pain signals in cell bodies of secondary sensory neurons in laminae I and II and transmit the outgoing nociceptive signals through axons forming the spinothalamic tract (7).

Descending inhibitory pathways

In addition to local modulation by interneurons, there are descending inhibitory pathways from the brain that also communicate with SCDH neurons through chemical signals. These include norepinephrine (NE), serotonin (5-HT), and endogenous opioids (see figure 2) (8).

Major noradrenergic inhibition originates at the locus coeruleus/subcoeruleus and travels to SCDH through the ventromedial funiculus. Evidence suggests that NE released from these inhibitory terminals acts through presynaptic α_2 receptors. Ligand binding of the presynaptic α_2 receptors induces the association of inhibitory G protein ($G_i/0$) with adenyl cyclase. As a result, adenyl cyclase is inactivated which results in a decrease of cyclic adenosine monophosphate (cAMP) production. This leads to a decrease of intracellular cAMP levels and protein kinase A phosphorylation to reduce presynaptic neurotransmitter release.Most SC serotoninergic inputs are from the nucleus raphe magnus in caudal brainstem. These fibers descend to SCDH to release 5-HT. At least 15 different 5-HT receptors, that mediate serotoninergic actions in SCDH during pain processing, are either facilitatory or inhibitory in pain processing (9). They are widely distributed throughout the nervous system, and their actions are usually mediated by G protein-coupled intracellular signaling events (9).

Endogenous opioids are expressed in the descending pathways originating from the periaqueductal gray in brainstem, and other related brain structures (10).

This pathway functions by activating opioid receptors on pre- and postsynaptic endings in SCDH neurons. Such receptors include mu (μ), delta (δ), and kappa (κ) opioid receptors, which have specific preferences for their endogenous ligands, including endorphins, dynorphins, and enkephalins (11, 12). Opioid receptors are widely distributed in the peripheral and central nervous systems to modulate nociception (13). Their activation by agonists is coupled with G protein G_i/G_0 which subsequently increases phosphodiesterase activity and inhibits neural membrane excitability and pain transmission.

Glutamate receptors

Most painful signals in the DH are mediated by glutamate, the most abundant excitatory amino acid in the central nervous system (CNS). Glutamate actions are mediated by several glutamate receptors: the α-amino-3-hydroxy-5-methyl-4-izoxazolepropionic acid receptors (AMPARs), the kainate receptors (KARs), and the N-methyl-D-aspartate receptors (NMDARs).

AMPARs are primary glutamate receptors that mediate nociception. They are ionotropic transmembrane molecules that mediate fast synaptic transmission in the central nervous system (CNS). AMPARs are composed of four types of subunits, designated as GluR1 through GluR4 (14, 15). Most consist of symmetric "dimers of dimers" of GluR1 and GluR2, GluR3, or GluR4 (16). AMPARs are rapid channels which open and close quickly following ligand binding. This feature results in rapid depolarization of the cell membrane without a long repolarization phase and thus renders the neuron able to respond to high-frequency stimulation. In fact, AMPARs mediate most of the fast excitatory synaptic transmissions in the CNS.

AMPARs that carry GluR2 subunits are sodium/potassium channels. The presence of GluR2 subunits inhibits calcium permeability of AMPARs (17). Since most AMPARs in the CNS have GluR2, AMPAR channel openings prevent inward calcium currents and protect neurons from calcium-mediated excitability (17).

KARs are glutamate receptors with selective affinity for their agonist, kainate. They mediate excitatory postsynaptic neurotransmission by binding glutamate but serve as presynaptic modulators to inhibit GABAergic neurons. Like AMPARs, KARs are located in both pre- and postsynaptic membranes and function as sodium/potassium channels (18). Compared with AMPARs, the repolarization phase of KARs takes longer, resulting in a slower response to high-frequency stimulation (18).

NMDARs are ionotropic glutamate receptors that selectively bind to NMDA. NMDARs are tetrameric ion channels consisting of two NR1 subunits in complex with two NR2 (A, B, C, and D subunits) or NR3 (A and B subunits) subunits (19). In addition, alternative splicing of the GluR1 subunit yields eight possible variants of this subunit. The NR1 subunit contains a binding site for glycine or D-serine, whereas the NR2 subunit contains the binding site for glutamate. In their quiescent state, NMDARs are blocked by Mg^{2+} ions. Opening of other ionotropic receptors, such as AMPARs, causes membrane depolarization. During this process, the Mg^{2+} blockade is removed and allows a voltage-dependent flow of Na^+ and Ca^{2+} ions into cells and K^+

out of cells. The NMDAR-dependent calcium influx triggers a series of signaling cascades that involve the activation of multiple protein kinases, including mitogen-activated protein kinase (MAPK) and protein kinase C (PKC) (20). This kinase activation further phosphorylates subunits of NMDARs and prolongs both channel opening and membrane depolarization. As a result of this unique feature, NMDARs mediate many biological functions including chronic pain, memory, and windup phenomenon (increased pain sensitivity after repeated stimuli) in distinct areas of the CNS (21).

Another glutamate receptor, metabotropic glutamate receptor (mGluR), also participates in pain processing. Unlike ionotropic glutamate receptors, mGluRs are coupled with G protein-dependent actions to trigger intracellular secondary messengers. MGluRs have 8 subtypes and many splice variant products. In general, mGluR1 and mGluR5 are better understood for pain processing compared to other isoforms. After noxious stimuli, these receptors respond to glutamate and activate phospholipase C /PKC pathways, which increase intracellular calcium levels (22).

Other neurotransmitters

Gamma-aminobutyric acid (GABA) is an inhibitory neurotransmitter that is affected after noxious stimuli. GABA acts through $GABA_A$ and $GABA_B$ receptors. Upon GABA binding, the $GABA_A$ receptors selectively open for Cl^- inflow and hyperpolarize the cell membrane of neurons. This causes an inhibitory effect on neurotransmission by blocking transmission of action potentials (23).

In contrast to the ionotropic $GABA_A$ receptors, the $GABA_B$ receptors are metabotropic transmembrane receptors. Through G-protein-coupled mechanisms, they open the K^+ channels and prevent cell membrane depolarization and action potential transmission.

In addition, $GABA_B$ receptors can also reduce activity of adenyl cyclase and decrease the cell's conductance to Ca^{2+}. Glycine is another major inhibitory neurotransmitter for modulating nociception. Actions of glycine are mediated by binding to glycine receptors (GlyR) that are distributed densely at superficial layers of the SCDH (24).

Neuropeptides

In painful states, afferent sensory fibers increase secretion of neuropeptides from their synapses with secondary neurons in the SCDH to mediate nociception. SP and CGRP are commonly associated with inflammatory and neuropathic models of pain. These neuropeptides are secreted from presynaptic terminals of Aδ and C fibers. They bind to their corresponding receptors (NK1 receptor for SP and CGRP receptor for CGRP) in both pre- and post-synaptic compartments in the SCDH. Other neuropeptides involved in nociception include cholecystokinin, neuropeptide Y, and bradykinin.

Spinal cord neural plasticity in chronic pain

There are several cellular and molecular mechanisms involved in the SC that are responsible for the development of chronic pain states:

1) Phenotype switch and neurotrophic factors. After peripheral painful stimulation, Aβ fibers, that normally do not process nociception, become sensitive to noxious stimuli. These large-diametered and myelinated sensory fibers conduct rapid nociceptive signals after inflammatory or neuropathic insults. In addition, they begin to express neuropeptides like SP and CGRP, as well as neurotrophic factors like brain-derived neurotrophic factor (BDNF) and NGF (25). NGF is produced in peripheral tissues and is retrogradely transported to DRG neurons. In DRG neurons, NGF binds to Trk A receptors and activates several protein kinases, including MAPK to upregulate expression of SP, CGRP, and BDNF that are then secreted into the DH by Trk A-positive afferent fibers. In the SCDH, most of BDNF's actions are mediated by the Trk B receptor. The action of BDNF binding to Trk B receptors induces the receptors' intrinsic tyrosine kinase activity, which in turn activates a series of downstream signaling events (26). As a result, peripheral sensory inputs to the SCDH are substantially increased and pain perception is therefore exaggerated. Since SP, CGRP, and BDNF expressions are dependent on NGF signaling, NGF is likely the key factor in this transformation of Aβ fibers.

2) Collateral sprouting. In painful conditions, nerve endings from Aβ afferents in the laminae III and IV of the SCDH could sprout and synapse with secondary neurons in laminae I and II. This phenomenon is associated with chemical factors generated in the superficial laminae with increased nociception (27). Potential causative factors include: (1) tumor necrosis factor-α (TNF-α) and cytokines released from activated microglia and astrocytes. These factors are known to stimulate neurotrophic factor expression which in turn could promote collateral sprouting in the DH (28). (2) BDNF released from NGF-positive primary afferents. BDNF has multiple effects on Trk B-expressing neurons to potentiate spinal nociceptive transmission, including stimulation of axon outgrowth and collateral sprouting (see Figure 3) (29).

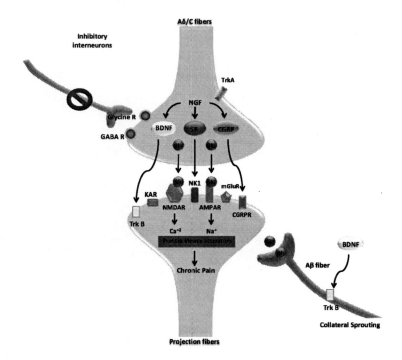

Figure 3. Spinal cord plasticity in chronic pain. In chronic pain, increased levels of neurotransmitters and neuropeptides induce postsynaptic hyperactivity in the second ordered neurons of the SCDH. As a result, the Mg^{+2} blockage of the NMDA receptor is removed, which causes the Ca^{+2} channel to open. As the channel opens, increased intracellular Ca^{+2} levels induces a series of downstream protein kinase phosphorylation, which in turn prolongs the depolarization of projection neurons to enhance nociception. In addition, collateral sprouting from Aβ fibers and decreased actions of local inhibitory interneurons further contribute to increased nociception.

3) Disinhibition. GABAergic and glycinergic interneurons of SCDH normally serve as presynaptic regulators for excessive nociception. However, this mechanism has a potential to become defective after nerve injury. In animal models of chronic pain, the numbers of GABA and glutamate decarboxylase (GAD)-positive interneurons are decreased due to apoptosis (30). This reduction of spinal inhibition results in hyperalgesia.

The actions of glycine receptors are also compromised during chronic pain. Prostaglandins released during chronic inflammatory conditions could deteriorate Glyrα3 function through EP2 receptors. This phenomenon is mediated by Gs protein and protein kinase A (Figure 3).

Other inhibitory systems involved in chronic pain include μ and δ-opioid receptors, α2-adrenergic receptor, purinergic A1 receptor, neuropeptide Y1 and Y2 receptors, cannabinoid CB1 and CB2 receptors, muscarinic M2 receptor, $GABA_B$ receptor, and somatostatin (31).

NMDA receptor activation

An essential step for augmented continuous pain is the activation of NMDA receptors on SCDH neurons. After repetitive, prolonged, or intense stimulation, membrane depolarization on postsynaptic terminals of secondary sensory neurons from AMPA, NK1, CGRPR currents release the Mg^{2+} blockade of NMDA receptors, which opens the ion channel. This causes a significant amount of Ca^{2+} inward current and triggers a series of intracellular reactions by activation of several intracellular protein kinases including protein kinase C and MAPK (Fig. 3) (20). In addition, increased intracellular Ca^{+2} levels trigger the activation of nitric oxide synthases (NOS) and cyclooxygenases (COX). As a consequence, enhanced channel conductance as well as receptor membrane trafficking contribute to prolonged membrane depolarization (1).

1) Other glutamate receptors. In painful conditions, increased peripheral afferent inputs induce a conversion from GluR2-containing AMPAR (impermeable to Ca^{2+}) to GluR1 (Ca^{2+} permeable) (32). This subunit switch of AMPARs affects AMPA-dependent intracellular signaling. In addition to Na^+ inflow after AMPA receptor activation, accompanied Ca^{2+} inward current triggers a wide variety of downstream intracellular activities, similar to NMDA receptor activation. This action further enhances response to painful stimuli in hyperalgesia. In addition to AMPAR, kainate receptors and mGluR5 contribute to chronic pain (33, 34).

2) Glial cell activation. After peripheral inflammatory reaction or nerve injury, SC glia are activated and contribute to enhanced neuronal excitability in the SCDH. Inflammatory mediators like SP, CGRP, nitric oxide (NO), adenosine-5'-triphosphate (ATP), tumor necrosis factors (TNFs), and prostaglandins (PGs) are upregulated in the periphery and transported into the SCDH. These agents activate glial cells, including microglia and astrocytes, to promote pain perception (Figure 4) (35).

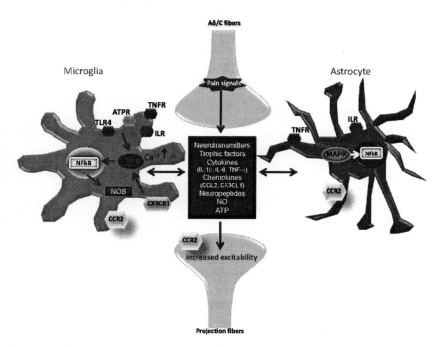

Figure 4. An activation of spinal glia in chronic pain. In chronic pain, increased levels of nociceptive mediators, including neurotransmitters, trophic factors, cytokines, chemokines, neuropeptides, NO, and ATP activate nearby astrocytes and microglia. These factors induce microglial p38 phosphorylation and nuclear translocation of NFκB in addition to promoting expression of cytokine, chemokine, and NO to the synaptic cleft. In addition, astrocytes respond to such mediators by similar actions through MAPK and NFκB activation. These inflammatory mediators bind to their corresponding receptors on neuronal and glial surfaces to further enhance the postsynaptic excitability of projection neurons. (TLR: toll-like receptors, ILR: interleukin receptors, TNFR: tumor necrosis factor receptors, ATPR: ATP receptors.).

Astrocytes are the most abundant glia in the CNS, and thus astrocytes have several important functions:

1) Astrocytes form the inner layer of the blood brain barrier.

Spinal cord neural plasticity in chronic pain ...

2) Astrocytes maintain the metabolic homeostasis of the CNS and regulate neuronal functions by reuptake of excess glutamate and GABA.
3) Astrocytes repair the nervous system after injury.

Astrocytes in the SCDH respond to painful stimuli by increasing their number and size. In addition, they express several proinflammatory cytokines, chemokines, and neurotrophic factors (35). After nerve injury, astrocytes increase their expression of interleukin (IL)-1β, and IL-6. Such upregulations are associated with the activation of nuclear factor of kappa light polypeptide gene enhancer in B-cells (NFκb) and MAPK signaling (36). These cytokines are secreted in the SCDH and stimulate postsynaptic neurons as well as nearby astrocytes and microglia. Likewise, chemokines like CCL2 and its receptor CCR2 are increased after nerve injury (35, 37, 38). These chemokines interact with their surface receptors on the neuronal terminals as well as other astrocytes and microglia (37). In the SCDH, chemokine signaling promotes intracellular activation of MAPK, including extracellular signal-regulated kinases (ERKs), p38, and c-Jun N-terminal kinases (JNKs), in addition to contributing to the enhancement of nociception (39). Additionally, astrocytes are important sources of BDNF in chronic pain models (35). BDNF binds to the postsynaptic Trk B receptor and promote intracellular signaling pathways, including MAPK activation.

Microglia make up 5% of the glial population. In the CNS, microglia serve as scavengers for the cell-mediated immune system. They respond to infections and tissue injury by releasing proinflammatory cytokines including interleukin-1β (IL-1β), IL-6, and TNF-α. After nerve injury, microglia are activated by several chemical factors including adenosine triphosphate (ATP) and nitric oxide. Increased ATP levels, due to nerve injury, trigger activation of microglial P2X4 receptors and induce cytokine expression through p38. Other ATP receptors (ATPR), including P2X3, P2X7 and P2Y12, are also involved in microglia-mediated chronic pain (40). Microglia also express chemokine receptors like CX3CL1 and CCR2, as well as respond to neuronal chemokines, such as CCL2, after nerve injury. These actions are believed to associate with allodynia following nerve injury (37). Like astrocytes, microglia secrete BDNF after nerve injury, a mechanism important for the plasticity of SCDH in chronic pain (41). Microglial BDNF signaling suppresses a Cl⁻ transporter (KCC2) and lowers the inhibitory actions of GABA receptors (42). Moreover, the signals from nerve injury also trigger the toll-like receptors (TLR) in microglia. This mechanism could contribute to opioid-induced side effects, which is frequently encountered in current practice (43).

Clinical implications

Currently, no treatment is available that targets phenotype switching in the development of chronic pain. Potential pharmacological approaches for inhibiting phenotype switch are:

1) Blocking neurotrophin signaling

Treatment approaches include anti-NGF and Trk A receptor blockade, which has been tested in clinical trials for treating chronic pain. A novel multipotent neurotrophin antagonist, 3-[(5E)-4-oxo-5-[[5-(4-sulfamoylphenyl)-2-furyl]methylene]-2-thioxo-thiazolidin-3-yl]propanoic acid (Y1036) has an affinity for both NGF and BDNF as well as prevents their binding to Trk A and Trk B receptors (44). In addition, inhibition of downstream signaling molecules, including MAPK, has proven to achieve analgesia in animal models (45).

2) Inhibiting SP and CGRP actions

There are currently several available treatments for chronic pain that inhibit SP and CGRP actions. Capsaicin, the spicy component of hot pepper, binds to the transient receptor potential vallinoid (TRPV)1 receptor and exhausts SP secretion to achieve analgesia (46). Gabapentin and pregabalin are blockers of a voltage gated calcium channel, $\alpha2\delta$. They decrease SC levels of neurotransmitters and neuropeptides, including SP and CGRP (47). Additionally, several NK1 antagonists have been tested in clinical trials for chronic pain. However, these compounds have not been successful in demonstrating analgesia (48). In contrast, a CGRPR antagonist, telcagepant (MK-0974), has shown efficacy against migraine (49).

Unfortunately, at this time, there are no available medications that block collateral sprouting. Based on the known mechanisms underlying collateral sprouting, inhibition of TNF-α, cytokines, and BDNF could be potential treatments to inhibit collateral sprouting after peripheral inflammation or nerve injury. In addition, NGF signaling blockade could also be a valuable approach since this treatment could result in dual action of pain control by decreasing the peripheral nociceptive inputs and eliminating the BDNF-mediated collateral sprouting in the SCDH. Currently, an anti-NGF antibody is under clinical trial for treating chronic pain.

Presently, several NMDA receptor antagonists are available such as dextromethorphan, which was tested for treatment of pain. Unfortunately, its efficacy is poor for analgesia and causes significant side effects (50). Memantin is a medication for Alzheimer's disease that blocks NMDARs. However, in most trials it has failed to demonstrate an analgesic action (50). Methadone is an opioid medication that has properties of NMDA blockade. Clinically, methadone is effective for treating multiple painful conditions. Its NMDA blockade is from d-methadone, one of the enantiomeric isoforms of methadone (51). In addition, bupivacaine, a local anesthetic that blocks sodium channels, blocks the NMDA receptor, an action which is independent of its sodium channel blockade (52). Ketamine, another anesthetic, is a potent NMDA receptor blocker. Unfortunately, it has significant side effects preventing long term use (53). Amantadine, another NMDAR antagonist, has little value for treating chronic pain (54).

There is no medication on the current market specifically targeting AMPARs. However, NS1290, an AMPAR blocker, has been tested in a clinical trial and shows promising results in treating chronic pain (55). Several antagonists are available for kainate receptors. These compounds are potent against chronic pain in a variety of animal models (56). Methylphenylethynylpyridine (MPEP) and its derivative, fenobam, are blockers for mGluR5 (34). Both demonstrate good analgesic actions against chronic pain in animal studies. However, these compounds have yet to pass clinical trials.

Current effective treatments for inhibiting glial actions in chronic pain are still lacking. Minocyclin, a tetracycline antibiotic, inhibits microglia activation in the SC in painful conditions. In addition, propentofylline, a methylxanthine derivative, exhibits anti-hyperalgesia by limiting microglial actions and reducing SC levels of IL-1β, IL-6, and TNF-α (57). AV411, a non-selective phosphodiesterase inhibitor, was found to suppress the expression of IL-1β, Il-6 and TNF-α in a rat model of paclitaxel-induced mechanical allodynia (58). Several inhibitors for p38 have been tested in clinical trials for chronic pain (59). Antagonizing ATP action is an effective approach for inhibiting glial action in chronic pain. Several antagonists for p2X3, p2X4, p2X7, and p2Y12 were reported to have promising analgesic efficacy in animal studies (40). All of the compounds have yet to be proven effective for treating chronic pain in clinical trials. In addition, several inhibitors for interleukins, TNF-α and their corresponding receptors, are available for treating inflammatory conditions (60). However, their roles for treating chronic pain are still unclear. CCR2 RA-[R] is a CCR2 antagonist that reduced neuropathic pain in animal models (61). Additionally, PF-4136309, another CCR2 antagonist, has been tested in a phase 2 clinical trial for treating chronic pain (38). In addition, inhibition of microglial TLR4 action could improve the utility of opioids by decreasing the unwanted side effects (43).

Descending inhibitory pathways control excessive nociception in normal conditions. They consist of pathways that expressed endogenous opioids, NE and 5-HT systems in the brain. To enhance the actions of opioid receptors in the CNS, opioids are frequently used to treat chronic pain from either inflammatory or neuropathic origins. Methadone, one of the synthetic opioids, inhibits activation of the NMDA receptor besides activating opioid receptors. Therefore, methadone is favored in treating chronic pain (51). In addition, several other treatment modalities that trigger production of endogenous opioids have been widely used for treating chronic pain. These treatments are transcutaneous electric stimulation, acupuncture, vagal stimulation, spinal cord and motor cortex stimulation (8).

For enhancing the NE inhibitory actions, α2 agonists are frequently used for chronic pain to inhibit presynaptic action potentials as well as enhance local GABAergic and glycinergic actions. In current practice, serotoninergic medications are widely used for chronic neuropathic pain, migraine, and fibromyalgia. Additionally, they are used for treating depression, which frequently is associated with chronic pain. However, specific serotonin reuptake inhibitors are not very effective for treating painful conditions. Medications like tricylic and tetracyclic antidepressants (TCAs) inhibit reuptakes of both 5-HT and NE and have been considered as the first line medication for neuropathic pain. Specific serotonin-norepinephrine reuptake inhibitors are more tolerable than TCAs and are frequently used for chronic pain by enhancing inhibitory actions from both systems.

It is a common practice to use GABAergic drugs for treating chronic pain. Benzodiazepines, agonists for the $GABA_A$ receptor, and baclofen, a $GABA_B$ receptor agonist, have been proven to have analgesic actions. In addition, α2 adrenoreceptor agonists (clonidine and tizanidine) could enhance GABAergic and glycinergic anti-nociception and have been applied for chronic painful conditions (62). By using a herpes simplex viral vector-mediated gene transfer for glutamic acid decarboxylase (GAD) local GABA levels in the SCDH increase, which could result in a potential treatment to enhance GABAergic action in the SCDH (63). Cyclooxygenase (COX) 1 and 2 inhibitors are potent medications for inhibiting PG production during inflammatory conditions. These medications could prevent inhibitory actions of PGs on Glyrα3 and preserve the glycinergic inhibition in the SCDH. However, COX inhibitors have been widely used for inflammatory pain from peripheral tissues. Their actions in the CNS are still unclear.

Conclusions

Chronic pain is a prevalent condition that causes significant burden on society. Increasing knowledge on the molecular mechanisms of chronic pain leads to the development of new treatments. Primary nociceptive inputs are modified within the SC through local and distant networks, and then are transmitted to higher levels of the nervous system. In this review, we focus on chronic pain-induced plasticity in SC neural circuits and their neurochemical properties. The change of neural circuits and neuron-glial interactions builds a strong foundation for the development of chronic pain. Understanding these processes has been a challenge for pain researchers. Although current mechanism-specific treatments for SC-mediated pain are limited, basic science research provides evidence to suggest potential new directions for treating chronic pain. However, most of these new treatments have not yet passed placebo-controlled clinical trials. As a result, more effort is urgently needed to develop mechanism-specific treatments for chronic pain.

Acknowledgment

The authors are supported by National Institutes of Health grant 1K08NS061039–01A2. No potential conflicts of interest relevant to this article were reported.

References

[1] Latremoliere A, Woolf CJ. Central sensitization: a generator of pain hypersensitivity by central neural plasticity. J Pain 2009;10(9):895-926.

[2]	Rexed B. The cytoarchitectonic organization of the spinal cord in the cat. J Comp Neurol 1952;96(3):414-95.
[3]	Todd AJ. Anatomy of primary afferents and projection neurones in the rat spinal dorsal horn with particular emphasis on substance P and the neurokinin 1 receptor. Exp Physiol 2002;87(2):245-9.
[4]	Lu Y, Perl ER. Modular organization of excitatory circuits between neurons of the spinal superficial dorsal horn (laminae I and II). J Neurosci 2005;25(15):3900-7.
[5]	Heinke B, Ruscheweyh R, Forsthuber L, Wunderbaldinger G, Sandkuhler J. Physiological, neurochemical and morphological properties of a subgroup of GABAergic spinal lamina II neurones identified by expression of green fluorescent protein in mice. J Physiol 2004;560(Pt 1):249-66.
[6]	Olave MJ, Puri N, Kerr R, Maxwell DJ. Myelinated and unmyelinated primary afferent axons form contacts with cholinergic interneurons in the spinal dorsal horn. Exp Brain Res 2002;145(4):448-56.
[7]	Braz JM, Nassar MA, Wood JN, Basbaum AI. Parallel "pain" pathways arise from subpopulations of primary afferent nociceptor. Neuron 2005;47(6):787-93.
[8]	Ren K aDR, Decending control mechanisms, In: Basbaum AI, Bushnell, M. C. Science of pain. San Diego: Elsevier, 2009:723-763.
[9]	Nichols DE, Nichols CD. Serotonin receptors. Chem Rev 2008;108(5):1614-41.
[10]	Copolov DL, Helme RD. Enkephalins and Endorphins. Clinical, pharmacological and therapeutic implications. Drugs 1983;26(6):503-19.
[11]	Fine PG, Portenoy RK, The Endogenous Opioid System. A Clinical Guide to Opioid Analgesia McGraw Hill, 2004.
[12]	Vanderah TW. Delta and kappa opioid receptors as suitable drug targets for pain. Clin J Pain 2010;26 Suppl 10(S10-5.
[13]	Stein C, Zollner C. Opioids and sensory nerves. Handb Exp Pharmacol 2009;194):495-518.
[14]	Song I, Huganir RL. Regulation of AMPA receptors during synaptic plasticity. Trends Neurosci 2002;25(11):578-88.
[15]	Mayer ML. Glutamate receptor ion channels. Curr Opin Neurobiol 2005;15(3):282-8.
[16]	Greger IH, Ziff EB, Penn AC. Molecular determinants of AMPA receptor subunit assembly. Trends Neurosci 2007;30(8):407-16.
[17]	Kim DY, Kim SH, Choi HB, Min C, Gwag BJ. High abundance of GluR1 mRNA and reduced Q/R editing of GluR2 mRNA in individual NADPH-diaphorase neurons. Mol Cell Neurosci 2001;17(6):1025-33.
[18]	Huettner JE. Kainate receptors and synaptic transmission. Prog Neurobiol 2003;70(5):387-407.
[19]	Paoletti P, Neyton J. NMDA receptor subunits: function and pharmacology. Curr Opin Pharmacol 2007;7(1):39-47.
[20]	Cheng HT, Suzuki M, Hegarty DM, Xu Q, Weyerbacher AR, South SM, Ohata M, Inturrisi CE. Inflammatory pain-induced signaling events following a conditional deletion of the N-methyl-D-aspartate receptor in spinal cord dorsal horn. Neuroscience 2008;155(3):948-58.

[21] Larsson M. Ionotropic glutamate receptors in spinal nociceptive processing. Mol Neurobiol 2009;40(3):260-88.

[22] Abe T, Sugihara H, Nawa H, Shigemoto R, Mizuno N, Nakanishi S. Molecular characterization of a novel metabotropic glutamate receptor mGluR5 coupled to inositol phosphate/Ca2+ signal transduction. J Biol Chem 1992;267(19):13361-8.

[23] Johnston GA. GABAA receptor pharmacology. Pharmacol Ther 1996;69(3):173-98.

[24] Zeihofer H, Glycine receptors, In: Basbaum A, Bushnell, MC. Science of Pain Elsevier, 2009:381-385.

[25] Cheng HT, Dauch JR, Hayes JM, Hong Y, Feldman EL. Nerve growth factor mediates mechanical allodynia in a mouse model of type 2 diabetes. J Neuropathol Exp Neurol 2009;68(11):1229-43.

[26] Pezet S, Malcangio M, Lever IJ, Perkinton MS, Thompson SW, Williams RJ, McMahon SB. Noxious stimulation induces Trk receptor and downstream ERK phosphorylation in spinal dorsal horn. Mol Cell Neurosci 2002;21(4):684-95.

[27] Mannion RJ, Doubell TP, Gill H, Woolf CJ. Deafferentation is insufficient to induce sprouting of A-fibre central terminals in the rat dorsal horn. J Comp Neurol 1998;393(2):135-44.

[28] Abe Y, Akeda K, An HS, Aoki Y, Pichika R, Muehleman C, Kimura T, Masuda K. Proinflammatory cytokines stimulate the expression of nerve growth factor by human intervertebral disc cells. Spine (Phila Pa 1976) 2007;32(6):635-42.

[29] Soril LJ, Ramer LM, McPhail LT, Kaan TK, Ramer MS. Spinal brain-derived neurotrophic factor governs neuroplasticity and recovery from cold-hypersensitivity following dorsal rhizotomy. Pain 2008;138(1):98-110.

[30] Eaton MJ, Plunkett JA, Karmally S, Martinez MA, Montanez K. Changes in GAD- and GABA- immunoreactivity in the spinal dorsal horn after peripheral nerve injury and promotion of recovery by lumbar transplant of immortalized serotonergic precursors. J Chem Neuroanat 1998;16(1):57-72.

[31] Taylor BK. Spinal inhibitory neurotransmission in neuropathic pain. Curr Pain Headache Rep 2009;13(3):208-14.

[32] Larsson M, Broman J. Translocation of GluR1-containing AMPA receptors to a spinal nociceptive synapse during acute noxious stimulation. J Neurosci 2008;28(28):7084-90.

[33] Wu LJ, Ko SW, Zhuo M. Kainate receptors and pain: from dorsal root ganglion to the anterior cingulate cortex. Curr Pharm Des 2007;13(15):1597-605.

[34] Montana MC, Cavallone LF, Stubbert KK, Stefanescu AD, Kharasch ED, Gereau RWt. The metabotropic glutamate receptor subtype 5 antagonist fenobam is analgesic and has improved in vivo selectivity compared with the prototypical antagonist 2-methyl-6-(phenylethynyl)-pyridine. J Pharmacol Exp Ther 2009;330(3):834-43.

[35] O'Callaghan JP, Miller DB. Spinal glia and chronic pain. Metabolism 2010;59 Suppl 1(S21-6.

[36] Milligan ED, Watkins LR. Pathological and protective roles of glia in chronic pain. Nat Rev Neurosci 2009;10(1):23-36.

[37] Abbadie C, Bhangoo S, De Koninck Y, Malcangio M, Melik-Parsadaniantz S, White FA. Chemokines and pain mechanisms. Brain Res Rev 2009;60(1):125-34.

[38] Gao YJ, Ji RR. Chemokines, neuronal-glial interactions, and central processing of neuropathic pain. Pharmacol Ther 2010;126(1):56-68.

[39] Gao YJ, Ji RR. Chemokines, neuronal-glial interactions, and central processing of neuropathic pain. Pharmacol Ther

[40] Jarvis MF. The neural-glial purinergic receptor ensemble in chronic pain states. Trends Neurosci 2010;33(1):48-57.

[41] Biggs JE, Lu VB, Stebbing MJ, Balasubramanyan S, Smith PA. Is BDNF sufficient for information transfer between microglia and dorsal horn neurons during the onset of central sensitization? Mol Pain 2010;6(44.

[42] Coull JA, Beggs S, Boudreau D, Boivin D, Tsuda M, Inoue K, Gravel C, Salter MW, De Koninck Y. BDNF from microglia causes the shift in neuronal anion gradient underlying neuropathic pain. Nature 2005;438(7070):1017-21.

[43] Watkins LR, Hutchinson MR, Rice KC, Maier SF. The "toll" of opioid-induced glial activation: improving the clinical efficacy of opioids by targeting glia. Trends Pharmacol Sci 2009;30(11):581-91.

[44] Eibl JK, Chapelsky SA, Ross GM. Multipotent neurotrophin antagonist targets brain-derived neurotrophic factor and nerve growth factor. J Pharmacol Exp Ther 2010;332(2):446-54.

[45] Ji RR, Gereau RWt, Malcangio M, Strichartz GR. MAP kinase and pain. Brain Res Rev 2009;60(1):135-48.

[46] Knotkova H, Pappagallo M, Szallasi A. Capsaicin (TRPV1 Agonist) therapy for pain relief: farewell or revival? Clin J Pain 2008;24(2):142-54.

[47] Fehrenbacher JC, Taylor CP, Vasko MR. Pregabalin and gabapentin reduce release of substance P and CGRP from rat spinal tissues only after inflammation or activation of protein kinase C. Pain 2003;105(1-2):133-41.

[48] Spath M. [What's new in the therapy of fibromyalgia?]. Schmerz 2003;17(6):437-40.

[49] Schelstraete C, Paemeleire K. CGRP antagonists: hope for a new era in acute migraine treatment. Acta Neurol Belg 2009;109(4):252-61.

[50] Sang CN, Booher S, Gilron I, Parada S, Max MB. Dextromethorphan and memantine in painful diabetic neuropathy and postherpetic neuralgia: efficacy and dose-response trials. Anesthesiology 2002;96(5):1053-61.

[51] Davis AM, Inturrisi CE. d-Methadone blocks morphine tolerance and N-methyl-D-aspartate-induced hyperalgesia. J Pharmacol Exp Ther 1999;289(2):1048-53.

[52] Furutani K, Ikoma M, Ishii H, Baba H, Kohno T. Bupivacaine Inhibits Glutamatergic Transmission in Spinal Dorsal Horn Neurons. Anesthesiology 2009;

[53] Cvrcek P. Side effects of ketamine in the long-term treatment of neuropathic pain. Pain Med 2008;9(2):253-7.

[54] Kavirajan H. Memantine: a comprehensive review of safety and efficacy. Expert Opin Drug Saf 2009;8(1):89-109.

[55] Gormsen L, Finnerup NB, Almqvist PM, Jensen TS. The efficacy of the AMPA receptor antagonist NS1209 and lidocaine in nerve injury pain: a randomized, double-blind, placebo-controlled, three-way crossover study. Anesth Analg 2009;108(4):1311-9.

[56] Ruscheweyh R, Sandkuhler J. Role of kainate receptors in nociception. Brain Res Brain Res Rev 2002;40(1-3):215-22.

[57] Whitehead KJ, Smith CG, Delaney SA, Curnow SJ, Salmon M, Hughes JP, Chessell IP. Dynamic regulation of spinal pro-inflammatory cytokine release in the rat in vivo following peripheral nerve injury. Brain Behav Immun 2009;

[58] Ledeboer A, Jekich BM, Sloane EM, Mahoney JH, Langer SJ, Milligan ED, Martin D, Maier SF, Johnson KW, Leinwand LA, Chavez RA, Watkins LR. Intrathecal interleukin-10 gene therapy attenuates paclitaxel-induced mechanical allodynia and proinflammatory cytokine expression in dorsal root ganglia in rats. Brain Behav Immun 2007;21(5):686-98.

[59] Coulthard LR, White DE, Jones DL, McDermott MF, Burchill SA. p38(MAPK): stress responses from molecular mechanisms to therapeutics. Trends Mol Med 2009;15(8):369-79.

[60] Kunz M, Ibrahim SM. Cytokines and cytokine profiles in human autoimmune diseases and animal models of autoimmunity. Mediators Inflamm 2009;2009(979258.

[61] Bhangoo S, Ren D, Miller RJ, Henry KJ, Lineswala J, Hamdouchi C, Li B, Monahan PE, Chan DM, Ripsch MS, White FA. Delayed functional expression of neuronal chemokine receptors following focal nerve demyelination in the rat: a mechanism for the development of chronic sensitization of peripheral nociceptors. Mol Pain 2007;3(38.

[62] Baba H, Goldstein PA, Okamoto M, Kohno T, Ataka T, Yoshimura M, Shimoji K. Norepinephrine facilitates inhibitory transmission in substantia gelatinosa of adult rat spinal cord (part 2): effects on somatodendritic sites of GABAergic neurons. Anesthesiology 2000;92(2):485-92.

[63] Wolfe D, Mata M, Fink DJ. A human trial of HSV-mediated gene transfer for the treatment of chronic pain. Gene Ther 2009;16(4):455-60.

Chapter IV

The role of neuroimaging in chronic pain syndromes

Christine Chang, MD[*1] *and Marco Pappagallo, MD*[2]
[1]Mount Sinai School of Medicine,
Department of Psychiatry, New York, New York, US
[2]Mount Sinai School of Medicine, Department of Anesthesiology,
New York, New York, US

Abstract

This chapter provides a broad overview of the higher brain structures involved in pain perception and modulation in chronic pain syndromes as revealed through neuroimaging. Further, this article highlights the findings of reviews and meta-analysis of neuroimaging in chronic pain, and focuses on the findings of cortical modulation of pain. Neuroimaging has significantly impacted chronic pain research and its potential to be used in clinical settings is discussed.

---

[*] Correspondence: Christine Chang, MD, Mount Sinai School of Medicine, Department of Psychiatry, One Gustave L Levy Place, New York, NY 10029 United States. E-mail: christine.m.chang@mssm.edu

Introduction

Chronic pain, a common medical problem affecting anywhere from 10 to 50 percent of the population, is understood to be a result of pathologic changes occurring on a hierarchy of levels within the central and peripheral nervous system (1). These changes encompass a range from the level of molecular (rNA and protein synthesis) to the structural (axonal sprouting, changes in brain volume) and may represent chronic pain as a disease state of "negative plasticity." That is, our brain's ability to change itself after injury, inflammation, or stress can be both positive and negative; in the case of chronic pain, the physical remapping has led to pain signals that continue when the initial injury has already resolved (1).

During the course of these dynamic changes, the central nervous system is continuously shaped by our multisensory experiences, such as attention, anticipation, emotion, and motivation (2-4). For instance, responses to stimuli are enhanced by directed attention to or negative anticipation of it (5-8) and emotions such as love can dull the pain from painful heat (9). Anticipation and negative anticipatory biases, such as fear, helplessness, or catastrophizing, may play an important role in the development and maintenance of chronic pain disorders as well as mood disorders (7).

These cognitive and affective components are recognized as part the experience of pain in addition to the more "objective" physiologic response to noxious stimuli (1,2, 10). Pain perception is regarded as the summation of different, partially independent pathways ascending in parallel from the spinal cord dorsal horn to the cortex (i.e. spinothalamic) sending pain signals from the periphery to the brain, while modulation is a descending, "top-down" pathway (1,2,11). The cognitive and affective experiences of pain have recently been demonstrated to have modulator influences as well; that is, areas in the brain that perceive pain can also "self-regulate" or modulate that experience (3-5,8,10-22). Both perception and modulation can undergo changes that lead to the development and pathology of chronic pain, and in recent years, pain modulation is increasingly being studied as a way to help patients control their own sensory experiences (23-32). The end result may be that was once told to patients as a symptom that was "all in their head" may actually be correctly identified to those areas of increased activity "in their head;" ideally, the patient may then be able to "rewire" their neural network.

This chapter highlights the recent groundbreaking work on the use of neuroimaging to study the brain's response to pain. Not only are cortical areas being identified in pain perception and modulation, but neuroimaging itself is being used in the modulation process (23). Neuroimaging has also shed light on the pathways of placebo and opioid analgesia (33), and many believe fMRI to be critical in the development of novel analgesics in the future (32-34).

The history of neuroimaging dates back to the early 1900s with a technique called pneumoencephalopathy (35). A form of magnetic resonance imaging (MRI) and computed tomography (CT) were developed in the 1970s and 1980s (35). However, it was with the development of functional neuroimaging in the last two decades that researchers are now able to directly observe cognitive activities, and under conditions of placebo, analgesia, directed tasks, and emotional states.

Currently, the types of neuroimaging are classically divided between two types: structural imaging, such as CT and MRI, which determines macroanatomic structure of the brain as well as tissue size and composition, and functional (PET, fMRI, SPECT, MEG) (32, 34-36). For chronic pain, much of the literature has been on the use of functional imaging techniques of PET and fMRI. PET scans detect pairs of gamma rays emitted indirectly by positron-emitting radionuclide (tracer), which is introduced into the body on a biologically active molecule. Images of tracer concentration within the body are then reconstructed by computer analysis. FMRI relies on the paramagnetic properties of oxygenated and deoxygenated hemoglobin to see images of changing blood flow in the brain associated with neural activity. This allows images to be generated that reflect which brain structures are activated (and how) during performance of different tasks (35, 36).

In a meta-analysis of the functional imaging of brain responses to pain, Peyron and colleagues found the following brain areas consistently activated by acute pain (37). The most consistently activated area across functional imaging studies was the insula and the secondary somatic regions (SII), followed by the anterior cingulated cortex (ACC), then followed less consistently by the contralateral thalamus and primary somatic cortex (SI). Regions activated in the attentional and affective components of pain were consistently the (mid) ACC, posterior parietal, and prefrontal cortices (37).

Peyron's review determined that, for response to noxious stimuli, "more than 50% of imaging studies have described a bilateral distribution of increased cerebral blood flow (CBF) in insular/SII cortices," citing 15 studies. However, it appeared that "insular activity is not related to attention. (37)" For the attentional, affective, and anticipation components of pain, Peyron breaks down reviews that localize these multisensory facets of pain into various parts of the anterior cingulated cortex. The ACC closely follows the anterior insula in the ranking of the most frequently reported site of regional CBF increase in pain, however its location of activation is complicated by what component of pain is being experienced. While most studies generally localize the emotional part of pain into the rostral ACC, and the cognitive into the middle ACC, these results are unclear. Peyron's meta-analyses concluded that the ACC supports multiple functions as a person experiences pain (37).

Peyron's meta-analysis supports the relatively recent understanding of the cortex being involved in pain modulation. The concept of pain modulation began with the gates theory (non-noxious input suppresses or closes the gate to noxious input at the spinal cord level) and is based physiologically on the finding that descending control of pain produces an analgesic effect (2-4,11). At all levels these ascending parts of the nociceptive system can be modulated by descending projections (pain modulation). The major brainstem regions that produce this effect were first located in poorly defined nuclei in the periaqueductal gray matter and the rostral medulla. However, current findings now demonstrate that higher brain structures than the PAG and medulla are potential sources of descending influence on nociceptive processes (1,3,4,11).

In addition to the meta-analysis by Peyron, other findings involving the ACC support the idea of cortical modulation of pain (10-22). Surgical lesions of the cingulated cortex and the neighboring white matter reduce the emotional value and the motivation to avoid painful stimuli but does not impair detection of painful stimuli. (38,39). Pain unpleasantness was also correlated with activity in the caudal ACC (4,24,25), with subjects reporting differing unpleasantness of pain but not intensity depending on ACC activity. Via hypnosis, researchers found significant modulation of dorsal ACC and prefrontal activity during noxious stimuli with no change in intensity of stimuli but reduced unpleasantness reported by subjects (24,25).

Within the ACC, there exist multiple areas for which the receiving and integration of attention, emotion, anticipation, and feeling are processed (10-22). It is also involved in autonomic regulation, and together with the function of selection and attention it does appear that the ACC is critical for "self-regulation of emotional responses" (3,4,7); hypnosis, biofeedback, directed attention, and anticipation, coping strategies have shown activity in the ACC that diminish the pain response, which would point towards the ACC being a part of the descending inhibitory pathways (24-30). Further support of the role of the ACC in modulating pain response is its activation under placebo analgesia. Recent functional imaging data provide evidence that the rostral ACC is a crucial cortical area for placebo analgesia and that this type of endogenous pain control depends on the enhanced functional connectivity of the rostral ACC with subcortical brain structures that are crucial for conditioned learning and descending inhibition of nociception. These results suggest that the ACC is involved in the transmission of pain sensation but also plays a role in processing pain-related emotion (11,40,41).

There is also a high level of opioid binding in the ACC (42), particularly the rostral ACC, and this endogenous opioid system may contribute to the placebo analgesia and pain modulation discussed above. One study demonstrated that the stronger placebo response a subject demonstrated, the more potent the mu opioid receptors were activated in the ACC, and the less the subjects reported pain. This further supports the endogenous opioid system in placebo analgesia with the ACC involved in descending inhibitory control (43).

The influence of mood and anxiety disorders, very frequently comorbid with chronic pain syndromes, on pain modulation is a complex topic; parts of the ACC share connections with areas implicated in emotional behavior such as the posterior orbital cortex, amygdala, hypothalamus, nucleus accumbens, periaqueductal grey area, ventral tegmental area, raphe nucleus, locus coeruleus, and nucleus tract solitarius (44). Current neuroimaging findings in major depressive disorder show the amygdala, areas of the ACC, and prefrontal cortex activated (7,44). In patients with MDD, depression symptom severity correlates with increased activity in the amygdala (44) and the amygdala is felt to be responsible for the "catastrophizing" and "helpnessness" feeling (7). Strigor found increased emotional reactivity to pain in patients with MDD and decreased modulation response compared to healthy controls, which he hypothesized could explain the "high comorbidity of pain and depression when the conditions become chronic (7)." Interestingly, treatment with antidepressants reverses the increased amygdala activity, demonstrating again the plasticity of the CNS (45-48).

Neuroimaging has significantly impacted our understanding of the sensation of pain, and allowed an anatomic framework for abstract concepts such as love, emotions, attention, fear, and anticipation. Cortical pathways involved in the perception and modulation of pain are increasingly being explored and understood. The plasticity of central nervous system as it relates to pain processing is further elucidated by neuroimaging studies demonstrating changes in activity in states of hypnosis, directed attention, concurrent psychiatric conditions, and even love Neuroimaging is likely to impact drug development in the future (32,34) , identifying drug responders versus non-responsders, revealing potential drug targets, as well as reducing the number of subjects needed with one subject allowed repeated scans (34). The potential for neuroimaging to teach "self-regulation" is still to be determined, though the idea is far-reaching; if patients can be taught to modulate their pain, the possibility exists that modulation of other neural pathways can occur.

References

[1] Merskey H, Bogduk N, eds. IASP Task Force on Taxonomy. Classification of chronic pain: Description of chronic pain syndromes and definition of pain terms. Seattle, WA: IASP Press, 1994.

[2] Price DD. Psychological and neural mechanisms of the affective dimension of pain. Science 2000;288:1769-72.

[3] Schnitzler A, Ploner M. Neurophysiology and functional neuroanatomy of pain perception. J Clin Neurophysiol 2000;17:592-600.

[4] Rainville P. Brain mechanisms of pain affect and pain modulation. Curr Opin Neurobiol 2002;12:195–204.

[5] Hsieh JC, Stone-Elander S, Ingvar M. Anticipatory coping of pain expressed in the human anterior cingulate cortex: a positron emission tomography study. Neurosci Lett 1999;262:61-4.

[6] Critchley HD, Mathias CJ, Dolan RJ. Neural activity in the human brain relating to uncertainty and arousal during anticipation. Neuron 2001;29:537-45.

[7] Strigo IA, Simmons AN, Matthews SC, Craig AD, Paulus MP. Association of major depressive disorder with altered functional brain response during anticipation and processing of heat pain. Arch Gen Psychiatry 2008;65:1275–84.

[8] Sawamoto N, Honda M, Okada T, et al. Expectation of pain enhances responses to nonpainful somatosensory stimulation in the anterior cingulate cortex and parietal operculum/posterior insula: an event-related functional magnetic resonance imaging study. J Neurosci 2000;20:7438-45.

[9] Younger J, Aron A, Parke S, Chatterjee N, Mackey S. Viewing Pictures of a Romantic Partner Reduces Experimental Pain: Involvement of Neural Reward Systems. PLoS ONE 5(10): e13309. doi:10.1371/journal.pone.0013309; 2010.

[10] Hutchison WD, Davis KD, Lozano AM, Tasker R, Dostrovsky JO. Pain-related neurons in the human cingulate cortex. Nat Neurosci 1999;2:403-5.

[11] Xie YQ, Huo FQ, Tang J.S. Cerebral cortex modulation of pain. Acta Pharmacologica Sinica, 2009;30(1):31.

[12] Ohara PT, Vit JP, Jasmin L. Cortical modulation of pain. Cell Mol Life Sci 2005; 62:44-52.

[13] Lenz FA, Rios M, Zirh A, Chau D, Krauss G, Lesser RP. Painful stimuli evoke potentials recorded over the human anterior cingulate gyrus. J Neurophysiol 1998; 79:2231-34.

[14] Bush G, Luu P, Posner MI. Cognitive and emotional influences in anterior cingulate cortex. Trends Cognit Sci 2000;4:215-22.

[15] Vogt BA, Sikes RW, Vogt LJ. Anterior cingulate cortex and the medial pain system. In: Vogt BA, Gabriel M, eds. Neurobiology of cingulate cortex and limbic thalamus: A comprehensive handbook. Boston, MA: Birkäuser, 1993:313-44.

[16] Davis KD, Taylor SJ, Crawley AP, Wood ML, Mikulis DJ. Functional MRI of pain- and attention-related activations in the human cingulate cortex. J Neurophysiol 1997;77:3370-80.

[17] Lane RD, Reiman EM, Axelrod B, Yun L-S, Holmes A, Schwartz GE. Neural correlates of levels of emotional awareness: evidence of an interaction between emotion and attention in the anterior cingulate cortex. J Cognit Neurosci 1998;10:525-35.

[18] Ploner M, Gross J, Timmermann L, Schnitzler A. Cortical representation of first and second pain sensation in humans. PNAS 2002;99:12444–8.

[19] Talbot JD, Marrett S, Evans AC, Meyer E, Bushnell MC, Duncan GH. Multiple representations of pain in human cerebral cortex. Science 1991;251:1355-8.

[20] Bush G, Luu P, Posner MI. Cognitive and emotional influences in anterior cingulate cortex. Trends Cognit Sci 2000;4:215-22.

[21] Rainville P, Duncan GH, Price DD, Carrier B, Bushnell MC. Pain affect encoded in human anterior cingulate but not somatosensory cortex. Science 1997;277:968-71.

[22] Hofbauer RK, Rainville P, Duncan GH, Bushnell MC. Cortical representation of the sensory dimension of pain. J Neurophysiol 2001;86:402-15.

[23] DeCharms RC, Maeda F, Glover GH, et al. Control over brain activation and pain learned by using real-time functional MRI. Proc Natl Acad Sci USA 2005;102(51):18626–31.

[24] Rainville P, Hofbauer RK, Paus T, Duncan GH, Bushnell MC, Price DD. Cerebral mechanisms of hypnotic induction and suggestion. J Cognit Neurosci 1999;11:110-25.

[25] Rainville P, Carrier B, Hofbauer RK, Bushnell MC, Duncan GH. Dissociation of pain sensory and affective dimensions using hypnotic modulation. Pain 1999;82:159-71.

[26] Wik G, Fisher H, Bragée B, Finer B, Fredrikson M. Functional anatomy of hypnotic analgesia: a PET study of patients with fibromyalgia. Eur J Pain 1999;3:7-12.

[27] Petrovic P, Petersson KM, Ghatan PH, Stone-Elander S, Ingvar M. Pain-related cerebral activation is altered by a distracting cognitive task. Pain 2000;85:19-30.

[28] Frankenstein UN, Richter W, McIntyre MC, Rémy F. Distraction modulates anterior cingulate gyrus activations during the cold pressor test. Neuroimage 2001;14:827–36.

[29] Seminowicz DA, Mikulis DJ, Davis KD. Cognitive modulation of pain-related brain responses depends on behavioral strategy. Pain 2004;112:48–58.

[30] Critchley HD, Melmed RN, Featherstone E, Mathias CJ, Dolan RJ. Brain activity during biofeedback relaxation: A functional neuroimaging investigation. Brain 2001;124:1003-12.

[31] Davis KD, Taylor SJ, Crawley AP, Wood ML, Mikulis DJ. Functional MRI of pain- and attention-related activations in the human cingulate cortex. J Neurophysiol 1997;77:3370-80.

[32] Borsook D, Moulton EA, Schmidt KF, Becerra LR. Neuroimaging revolutionizes therapeutic approaches to chronic pain. Mol Pain. 2007;3:25.

[33] Petrovic P, Kalso E, Petersson KM, Ingvar M. Placebo and opioid analgesia — imaging a shared neuronal network. Science 2002;295:1737-40.

[34] Lawrence J, Mackey SC. Role of neuroimaging in analgesic drug development. Drugs RD 2008;9(5):323-34.
[35] Beaumont, J. Graham. Introduction to Neuropsychology. New York: Guilford, 1983.
[36] Raichle ME, Mintun MA. Brain work and brain imaging. Ann Rev Neurosci 2006 29:449-76.
[37] Peyron R, Laurent B, Garcia-Larrea L. Functional imaging of brain responses to pain. A review and meta-analysis. Neurophysiol Clin 2000;30:263-88.
[38] Hurt RW, Ballantine HT. Stereotactic anterior cingulate lesions for persistent pain: a report of 68 cases. Clin Neurosurg 1973;21:334-51.
[39] Folz EL, White LE. Pain "relief" by frontal cingulotomy. J Neurosurg 1962;19:89-100.
[40] Amanzio M, Pollo A, Benedetti F. Endogenous opioids mediate both placebo analgesia and placebo respiratory depression. Soc Neurosci Abstr 1998;495.11.
[41] Bingel U, Lorenz J, Schoell E, Weiller C, Buchel C. Mechanisms of placebo analgesia: rACC recruitment of a subcortical antinociceptive network. Pain 2006;120:8–15.
[42] Jones AK, Qi LY, Fujirawa T, et al. In vivo distribution of opioid receptors in man in relation to the cortical projections of the medial and lateral pain systems measured with positron emission tomography. Neurosci Lett 1991;126: 25–8.
[43] Zubieta JK, Smith YR, Bueller J, et al. Regional opioid receptor regulation of sensory and affective dimensions of pain. Science 2001;293:311-5.
[44] Drevets WC. Neuroimaging and neuropathological studies of depression: Implications for the cognitive-emotional features of mood disorders. Curr Opin Neurobiol 2001;11(2):240-9.
[45] Harmer CJ, Mackay CE, Reid CB, et al. Antidepressant drug treatment modifies the neural processing of nonconscious threat cues. Biol Psychiatry 2006;59:816–20.
[46] Drevets WC. Neuroimaging abnormalities in the amygdala in mood disorders. Ann N Y Acad Sci 2003;985:420–44.
[47] Norbury R, Mackay CE. Short-term antidepressant treatment and facial processing:Functional magnetic resonance imaging study. Br J Psychiatry 2007;190:531–2.
[48] Walsh ND, Williams SC, Brammer MJ, et al. A longitudinal functional magnetic resonance imaging study of verbal working memory in depression after antidepressant therapy. Biol Psychiatr 2007;62:1236–43.

Chapter V

Sensorimotor training and its implication for cortical reorganization

Martin Diers, PhD, MSc and Herta Flor, PhD, MSc[*]
Department of Cognitive and Clinical Neuroscience,
Central Institute of Mental Health,
University of Heidelberg, Mannheim, Germany

Abstract

Several disorders that involve motor and sensory disturbances such as chronic pain, tinnitus or stroke are also characterized by changes in the sensory and motor maps in the sensorimotor cortices. This chapter reviews training procedures that target these maladaptive changes in states of chronic pain and the behavioral and cortical changes that accompany them. In addition, we will discuss factors that influence training success and discuss new developments. These procedures include training of perceptual abilities, motor function, and direct cortical stimulation and have been shown to reorganize the altered sensory and motor maps. Treatments that combine several modalities such as imagery

---

[*] Correspondence: Martin Diers or Herta Flor, Department of Cognitive and Clinical Neuroscience, Central Institute of Mental Health, University of Heidelberg, Square J5, D-68159 Mannheim, Germany. E-mail: martin.diers@zi-mannheim.de, herta.flor@zi-mannheim.de

or mirror treatment as well as use of prostheses also have beneficial effects. Further research must elucidate the mechanisms of these plastic changes related to the disorders and treatments.

Introduction

An injury- or stimulation-related increase or decrease of sensory input into the brain leads to changes in the respective primary sensory and usually also the motor areas and these alterations can be associated with unpleasant sensations such as pain. In these disorders sensory or motor training seems to be useful and is increasingly employed. In this review we will focus on sensorimotor training in states of chronic pain such as phantom limb pain, complex regional pain syndrome or chronic back pain. First, we will briefly describe cortical changes that are characteristic for these disorders and will then discuss sensorimotor training including stimulation methods and will focus on their effects, potential mechanisms and future developments.

Recovery of function is based on two mechanisms: compensatory processes and restitution (for a review see 1) and it is likely that both occur simultaneously in many cases. Compensatory processes are described as functional reorganization or functional adaptation and are achieved largely by the reorganization of surviving neural circuits to enable a given behavior over different circuits (2). Training leads to a redistribution of representations to non-damaged areas of sensory cortex via reorganization (3). By partial restitution of the impaired neuropsychological processes themselves on the basis of experience-dependent brain plasticity the formerly used brain circuits will reconstitute. Plastic reorganization can occur through two types of processes: First, an alteration in synaptic sensitivity related to unmasking of existing connections through change in the inhibitory dynamics. In contrast to structural changes which take days and weeks to develop, this happens in seconds to minutes (4). Second, the reduced level of activity in the area of the lesion weakens the synaptic connections between the damaged and undamaged sites leading to a reduced synchronous firing of cells in these two areas and thus weakening synaptic connectivity between them. This loss of connectivity results in depression of function in the structurally undamaged but functionally partly disconnected site. In some types of chronic pain such as chronic musculoskeletal pain syndromes an expansion of cortical representation zones and enhanced excitability and activation rather than a loss of injury-related function can be observed (5-9). Here enhanced input may lead to Hebbian learning and subsequent stimulation-induced plasticity (10, 11). A number of different approaches such as stimulation, bottom-up targeted stimulation, top-down targeted stimulation, manipulation of inhibitory processes, and manipulation of arousal mechanisms can be derived from these processes.

Neuropathic pain

Injury-related brain changes

In persons with amputations it has been shown that the region of the somatosensory cortex that formerly received input from the now amputated limb reorganizes and receives input from neighboring regions (12-14). These changes are mirrored in motor cortex (15-18). Interestingly, reorganizational changes were only found in amputees with phantom limb pain after amputation, but not in amputees without pain. This suggests that pain may contribute to the changes observed and that the persisting pain might also be a consequence of the plastic changes that occur. In several studies carried out on human upper-extremity amputee patients, displacement of the lip representation in the primary motor and somatosensory cortex was positively correlated with the intensity of phantom limb pain, and was not present in pain-free amputee patients or healthy control subjects. In addition, in the patients with phantom limb pain, but not in the pain-free amputee patients, imagined movement of the phantom hand was shown to activate the neighboring face area (18). This co-activation probably occurs due to the high overlap of the hand, arm, and mouth representations.

Similar observations have been made in patients with complex regional pain syndrome (CRPS). In these patients, the representation of the affected hand tended to be smaller compared with that of the unaffected hand and the individual digit representations had moved closer together (19-23). The extent of the pathological changes in the cortical representations correlated with the intensity of pain or motor dysfunction (21, 24, 25), but was additionally related to a degradation of sensibility in the affected hand. It was, however, unrelated to a loss of motor function (25). It is so far not known how an expansion of adjacent representations and a shrinking of adjacent representations as observed in phantom limb pain and CRPS, respectively, can both be associated with pain. However, it is possible that a degradation of the representations resembles a reduction of representational areas whereas an expansion and overlap is visible as enlargement.

Sensory and motor training

In amputees with phantom pain, several stimulation-related procedures were found to be effective. Intense input into the cortical amputation zone by the use of a myoelectric prosthesis or other prosthetic devices, for example, was found to reduce both cortical reorganization and phantom limb pain (26, 27). In patients in whom the use of prosthesis is not possible, sensory discrimination training might be beneficial. In one study, electrodes were closely spaced over the amputation stump in a region where stimulation excites the nerve that supplies the amputated portion of the arm. Patients then had to discriminate the frequency and location of the stimulation in an extended training period that lasted 90 min/day over a 2-week period. Substantial improvements to both two-point discrimination and phantom limb pain were demonstrated in the trained patients. These improvements were accompanied by changes in cortical reorganization, indicating a normalization of the shifted mouth representation (28). An asynchronous stimulation of the stump and lip area also yielded a significant reduction in phantom limb pain suggesting that the separation of overlapping cortical networks involved in pain may be important (29).

Similar results were found in CRPS patients where active discrimination between tactile stimuli led to an improvement in pain intensity and two point discrimination compared to passive stimulation alone (30). When patients watch the reflected image of their unaffected limb during training the effect of tactile discrimination training is enhanced (31). Tactile spatial acuity also improved when a Hebbian stimulation protocol of tactile coactivation (32) was used. The question arises if active stimulation is necessary or if passive stimulation is sufficient. In rats it could be shown that associative (Hebbian) pairing of passive tactile stimulation leads to a selective enlargement of the areas of cortical neurons representing the stimulated skin fields and of the corresponding receptive fields (11). In humans paired tactile stimulation goes along with an improved spatial discrimination performance (11, 33) matched by alterations of primary somatosensory cortex (34) indicating that fast plastic processes based on co-activation patterns act on a cortical and perceptual level. It is possible that in healthy controls passive stimulation without a task is sufficient for changes on the perceptual and cortical level whereas patients, who are less able to discriminate stimuli (30, 32), may need active stimulation for an improvement in discrimination ability (and pain intensity). These training effects can be enhanced by the use of pharmacological agents. For example, two-point discrimination after a coactivation protocol was doubled by amphetamine and was blocked by a N-methyl-D-aspartate-receptor blocker (35), or Lorazepam, a GABAA receptor agonist (36). However, these pharmacological modulation effects are not easily translated into clinical practice. In stroke patients amphetamine showed mixed results (37).

Mirror and motor imagery training

Ramachandran et al. (38) suggested that the use of a mirror might reverse the reorganizational changes observed in patients with phantom limb pain and they provided anecdotal evidence that viewing movements of one's intact hand in a mirror, which provides the impression of viewing the amputated hand, led to better movement of and less pain in the phantom limb. In lower limb amputees Brodie (39) reported a significantly greater number of movements in the phantom when a mirror box was used. Hunter et al. (40) showed that a single trial mirror box intervention led to a more vivid awareness of the phantom and a new or enhanced ability to move the phantom. Contrasting a mirror box with executed movement Brodie et al. (41) reported that movements in front of a mirror as well as movements without a mirror attenuated phantom limb pain and phantom sensation. Contrary to these findings, which were based on a single trial, 4 weeks of mirror training led to significantly more decrease in phantom limb pain than training with a covered mirror or using mental visualization in lower limb amputees (42) suggesting that phantom pain can be altered by visual feedback. It is well known that vision tends to take precedence over the other senses (touch included) when conflicting information is presented to vision and another sense (30, 43, 44). We recently observed in an fMRI session that amputees with phantom limb pain were unable to activate the sensorimotor cortex opposite to the amputated limb when the intact hand was moved in front of a mirror (appearing as movement of the phantom). A similar lack of activation was, however, also present with executed movements of the intact hand and with imagery of the phantom hand (45). Moreover, phantom limb pain was inversely correlated with activation on the hemisphere contralateral to the amputation suggesting that mirror training may not be special (46).

Other reports on imagined phantom movements in amputees (18, 47-50) showed activation in primary sensorimotor cortex representing the amputated limb in the pain free amputees and the healthy controls but not in the patients with phantom limb pain (45) and were supported by results from transcranial magnetic stimulation (TMS), which showed that perceived phantom hand movement could be triggered by stimulation over the motor cortex in an area that represented the now amputated limb (51). Both Giraux and Sirigu (52) and MacIver and colleagues (53) showed that imagery alone also affects the cortical map representing the amputated limb and relieves phantom limb pain in contrast to Chan and colleagues (42) who did not find changes in phantom pain related to imagery but did not assess cortical changes. These studies suggest that several types of modification of input into the affected brain region may alter pain sensation (see MacIver and colleagues, in this issue).

Moseley used a tripartite program to treat patients with CRPS (54, 55). This program consisted of: a hand laterality recognition task (a pictured hand was to be recognized as left or right); imagined movements of the affected hand; and mirror therapy (patients were asked to adopt the hand posture of both hands shown on a picture in a mirror box while watching the reflection of the unaffected hand). After a 2-week treatment, pain scores were found to be significantly reduced. They replicated this result in CRPS and phantom limb pain patients (56). In addition, McCabe and colleagues (57) found a reduction in pain ratings during and after mirrored visual feedback of movement of the unaffected limb in CRPS patients. Gieteling and colleagues (58) asked CRPS patients with dystonic postures of the right upper extremity to execute or imagine movements during a functional magnetic resonance (fMRI) measurement. Compared with controls, imaginary movement of the affected hand in patients showed reduced activation in the ipsilateral premotor and adjacent prefrontal cortex, and in a cluster comprising the frontal operculum, the anterior part of the insular cortex and the superior temporal gyrus. On the contralateral side, reduced activation was seen in the inferior parietal and adjacent primary sensory cortex. There were no differences between patients and controls when they executed movements, nor when they imagined moving their unaffected hand. Transcranial motor cortex stimulation has also been employed successfully for CRPS (e.g., 59).

Until now only little research has focused on mirror training, distorted body image and cortical representations in chronic musculoskeletal pain. A recent study suggeste the use of mirror training to treat fibromyalgia and found anecdotal evidence for reduced pain ratings (60). In chronic back pain a disrupted body image and decreased tactile acuity, measured by two-point discrimination, in the area of usual pain was found (61). Patients in this study reported that they could not find the outline of their trunk in the region of chronic pain. In another study, patients with chronic back pain participated on a left/right trunk rotation judgment task and a left/right hand judgment (62). The patients made more mistakes and were less accurate in the trunk rotation task. No differences were found for the hand judgment task. This gives further evidence of a disrupted working body schema of the trunk in this patient population. In these disorders another kind of visual feedback is used in behavioral treatments that focus on the exticntion of pain behaviors and the acquisition of healthy behaviors. There video feedback of patients' pain behaviorsand activity trainings as well as spouse trainings are used is used to extinguish pain and to increase helathy behaviors with concomitant positive brain changes (63, 64).

Virtual reality approaches to mirror training and robotic applications

Using a mirror box has some technical limitations. The intact limb has to move symmetrically with the mirrored limb. This is especially highly unnatural for the leg. This led to the invention of virtual reality (VR) and augmented reality (AR) mirror boxes (for a review see 65). In a first approach the perceived phantom arm was presented on a flat screen in 3D and controlled via a wireless data glove on the intact arm (66). The advantage of the VR mirror box was the possibility of incongruent movements between the intact hand with the data glove and the virtual phantom hand. For example, some of the virtual/phantom fingers were frozen and movements of the complete phantom led to more pain. The number of moved phantom fingers was thus gradually increased and it came to a relaxation and less pain sensation in 2 of the 3 cases. A different approach used immersive virtual reality (IVR) to transpose the movements made by an amputee's remaining anatomical limb into movements of a virtual limb (67). These authors found a reduction of phantom pain intensity in 2 of 3 cases (68, 69). The advantage of this system is that the entire body is implemented in the IVR and thus complex hand-eye coordination is possible. A novel variation on this method is using motion capture to collect data directly from a patient's stump and then transform it into goal directed, virtual action in the VR environment (70). In a first experimental study with 14 patients 72 % reported the ability to move the phantom and a reduction in phantom limb pain. These virtual reality applications are promising and could be extended in the future. With the rubber hand illusion it could be shown that the transfer of tactile sensations from the stump to a prosthetic limb by tricking the brain is possible (71). This is an important contribution to the field of neuroprosthetics where a major goal is to develop artificial limbs that feel like a real part of the body. Another possibility is a flexible multielectrode implantation for multi-movement prosthesis control and sensory feedback. The multielectrodes were implanted in the median and ulnar nerves of an amputee and led to real-time control of motor output (72).

Direct brain stimulation methods

Transcranial motor cortex stimulation (TMS) alters cortical excitability changes in the human brain noninvasively over a long time. It induces a facilitatory or inhibitory effect on corticospinal and cortico-cortical excitability. Repetitive TMS (rTMS) contralateral to the CRPS-affected side has also been employed successfully for CRPS (59). Pain relief occurred 30 s after stimulation, whereas the maximum effect was found 15 min later. Pain re-intensified increasingly 45 min after rTMS. In chronic back pain patients 20 Hz rTMS over the motor cortex decreases detection and pain thresholds for cold and heat sensations (73). In fibromyalgia syndrome rTMS over the right dorsolateral prefrontal cortex led to an improvement of pain (74).

An alternative method to induce neuroplastic changes is transcranial direct current stimulation (tDCS), which has its effect primarily on the membrane potential, by hyperpolarizing or depolarizing it. Transcranial direct current stimulation (tDCS) with the anode centered over M1 (2 mA, 20 minutes for five consecutive days) increased sleep efficiency (75) and decreased pain associated with an improvement in fibromyalgia symptoms (as indexed by the Fibromyalgia Impact Questionnaire) (76). Five daily sessions of 20 minutes of 1 mA tDCS over the hand area in the motor cortex produced long-lasting pain relief in patients with chronic pain such as back pain, fibromyalgia, poststroke pain syndrome, trigeminal neuralgia (59, 73). For a review of TMS (77), rTMS and tDCS interventions in chronic pain see (59, 73).

Discussion

Based on neuroscientific evidence on alterations in the primary sensory and motor areas in sensory and motor disorders such as chronic pain sensory and motor training methods have been developed. They include training of perceptual abilities, motor function, direct cortical stimulation as well as behavioral approaches and have been shown to reorganize altered sensory and motor maps. The cellular mechanisms underlying these changes still need to be determined but they involve changes in inhibitory circuits and long term synaptic changes. In addition, treatments that combine several modalities such as imagery or mirror treatment as well as use of prostheses seem to have beneficial effects. Direct brain stimulation methods such as TMS or tDCS have also been employed successfully in these disorders. This review has several limitations. First, we have only discussed a selected group of disorders where cortical reorganization occurs. Second, we have only described these changes in humans and have focused on implications for treatment rather than explaining mechanisms. Third, we have not been exhaustive with respect to the stimulation-related approaches but have only described exemplary results. For more comprehensive reviews see (78). Finally, much work still needs to be done to demonstrate the efficacy of these plasticity-related treatment approaches, which were usually tested in small heterogeneous samples without adequate controls and without adequate follow-ups. However, they may point out new approaches to treatment of chronic disorders and rehabilitation for the future. Future research should explore additional benefits which might arise from using brain stimulation methods in conjunction with behavioral trainings, virtual reality applications or plasticity-modifying pharmacological interventions.

Acknowledgment

The completion of this article was facilitated by the Bundesministerium für Bildung und Forschung (01EM0512, German Research Network on Neuropathic Pain, DFNS), and The State of Baden-Württemberg Research Prize. Further on support of this study was provided by the SOMAPS project, which receives research funding from the European Community's Sixth Framework Programme (FP6-NEST 043432 SOMAPS) and the PHANTOMMIND project, which receives research funding from the European Community's Seventh Framework Programme (FP7/2007-2013) / ERC grant agreement n° 230249. This manuscript reflects only the author's views and the Community is not liable for any use that may be made of the information contained therein.

References

[1] Robertson IH, Murre JM. Rehabilitation of brain damage: brain plasticity and principles of guided recovery. Psychol Bull 1999;125(5):544-75.

[2] Luria AR. Restoration of function after brain injury. Oxford, England: Pergamon; 1973.

[3] Xerri C, Merzenich MM, Peterson BE, Jenkins W. Plasticity of primary somatosensory cortex paralleling sensorimotor skill recovery from stroke in adult monkeys. J Neurophysiol 1998;79(4):2119-48.

[4] Donoghue JP. Plasticity of adult sensorimotor representations. Curr Opin Neurobiol 1995;5(6):749-54.

[5] Flor H, Braun C, Elbert T, Birbaumer N. Extensive reorganization of primary somatosensory cortex in chronic back pain patients. Neurosci Lett 1997;224(1):5-8.

[6] Gracely RH, Petzke F, Wolf JM, Clauw DJ. Functional magnetic resonance imaging evidence of augmented pain processing in fibromyalgia. Arthritis Rheum 2002;46(5):1333-43.

[7] Giesecke T, Gracely RH, Grant MA, Nachemson A, Petzke F, Williams DA, et al. Evidence of augmented central pain processing in idiopathic chronic low back pain. Arthritis Rheum 2004;50(2):613-23.

[8] Cook DB, Lange G, Ciccone DS, Liu WC, Steffener J, Natelson BH. Functional imaging of pain in patients with primary fibromyalgia. J Rheumatol 2004;31(2):364-78.

[9] Jensen KB, Petzke F, Carville S, Fransson P, Marcus H, Williams SC, et al. Anxiety and depressive symptoms in Fibromyalgia are related to low health esteem but not to pain sensitivity or cerebral processing of pain. Arthritis Rheum 2010.

[10] Recanzone GH, Schreiner CE, Merzenich MM. Plasticity in the frequency representation of primary auditory cortex following discrimination training in adult owl monkeys. J Neurosci 1993;13(1):87-103.

[11] Godde B, Spengler F, Dinse HR. Associative pairing of tactile stimulation induces somatosensory cortical reorganization in rats and humans. Neuroreport 1996;8(1):281-5.

[12] Elbert TR, Flor H, Birbaumer N, Knecht S, Hampson S, Larbig W, et al. Extensive reorganization of the somatosensory cortex in adult humans after nervous system injury. Neuroreport 1994;5:2593-2597.

[13] Yang TT, Gallen C, Schwartz B, Bloom FE, Ramachandran VS, Cobb S. Sensory maps in the human brain. Nature 1994;368(6472):592-3.

[14] Flor H, Elbert T, Knecht S, Wienbruch C, Pantev C, Birbaumer N, et al. Phantom-limb pain as a perceptual correlate of cortical reorganization following arm amputation. Nature 1995;375(6531):482-484.

[15] Cohen LG, Bandinelli S, Findley TW, Hallett M. Motor reorganization after upper limb amputation in man. Brain 1991;114:615-627.

[16] Kew JJ, Ridding MC, Rothwell JC, Passingham RE, Leigh PN, Sooriakumaran S, et al. Reorganization of cortical blood flow and transcranial magnetic stimulation maps in human subjects after upper limb amputation. J Neurophysiol 1994;72(5):2517-24.

Sensorimotor training and its implication for cortical reorganization 87

[17] Karl A, Birbaumer N, Lutzenberger W, Cohen LG, Flor H. Reorganization of motor and somatosensory cortex in upper extremity amputees with phantom limb pain. The Journal of Neuroscience 2001;21(10):3609-3618.

[18] Lotze M, Flor H, Grodd W, Larbig W, Birbaumer N. Phantom movements and pain. An fMRI study in upper limb amputees. Brain 2001;124:2268-2277.

[19] Juottonen K, Gockel M, Silen T, Hurri H, Hari R, Forss N. Altered central sensorimotor processing in patients with complex regional pain syndrome. Pain 2002;98(3):315-23.

[20] Schwenkreis P, Janssen F, Rommel O, Pleger B, Volker B, Hosbach I, et al. Bilateral motor cortex disinhibition in complex regional pain syndrome (CRPS) type I of the hand. Neurology 2003;61(4):515-9.

[21] Pleger B, Tegenthoff M, Ragert P, Forster AF, Dinse HR, Schwenkreis P, et al. Sensorimotor retuning [corrected] in complex regional pain syndrome parallels pain reduction. Ann Neurol 2005;57(3):425-9.

[22] Maihöfner C, Handwerker HO, Neundorfer B, Birklein F. Patterns of cortical reorganization in complex regional pain syndrome. Neurology 2003;61(12):1707-15.

[23] Maihöfner C, Handwerker HO, Birklein F. Functional imaging of allodynia in complex regional pain syndrome. Neurology 2006;66(5):711-7.

[24] Maihöfner C, Handwerker HO, Neundorfer B, Birklein F. Cortical reorganization during recovery from complex regional pain syndrome. Neurology 2004;63(4):693-701.

[25] Maihöfner C, Baron R, DeCol R, Binder A, Birklein F, Deuschl G, et al. The motor system shows adaptive changes in complex regional pain syndrome. Brain 2007;130(Pt 10):2671-87.

[26] Weiss T, Miltner WH, Adler T, Bruckner L, Taub E. Decrease in phantom limb pain associated with prosthesis-induced increased use of an amputation stump in humans. Neurosci Lett 1999;272(2):131-4.

[27] Lotze M, Grodd W, Birbaumer N, Erb M, Huse E, Flor H. Does use of a myoelectric prostesis prevent cortical reorganisation and phantom limb pain? Nature Neuroscience 1999;2(6):501-502.

[28] Flor H, Denke C, Schaefer M, Grüsser S. Effect of sensory discrimination training on cortical reorganisation and phantom limb pain. The Lancet 2001;375:1763-1764.

[29] Huse E, Preissl H, Larbig W, Birbaumer N. Phantom limb pain. Lancet 2001;358(9286):1015.

[30] Moseley GL, Zalucki NM, Wiech K. Tactile discrimination, but not tactile stimulation alone, reduces chronic limb pain. Pain 2008;137(3):600-8.

[31] Moseley GL, Wiech K. The effect of tactile discrimination training is enhanced when patients watch the reflected image of their unaffected limb during training. Pain 2009;144(3):314-9.

[32] Maihöfner C, DeCol R. Decreased perceptual learning ability in complex regional pain syndrome. Eur J Pain 2007;11(8):903-9.

[33] Godde B, Stauffenberg B, Spengler F, Dinse HR. Tactile coactivation-induced changes in spatial discrimination performance. J Neurosci 2000;20(4):1597-604.

[34] Godde B, Ehrhardt J, Braun C. Behavioral significance of input-dependent plasticity of human somatosensory cortex. Neuroreport 2003;14(4):543-6.

[35] Dinse HR, Ragert P, Pleger B, Schwenkreis P, Tegenthoff M. Pharmacological modulation of perceptual learning and associated cortical reorganization. Science 2003;301(5629):91-4.

[36] Dinse HR, Ragert P, Pleger B, Schwenkreis P, Tegenthoff M. GABAergic mechanisms gate tactile discrimination learning. Neuroreport 2003;14(13):1747-51.

[37] Carter AR, Connor LT, Dromerick AW. Rehabilitation after stroke: current state of the science. Curr Neurol Neurosci Rep;10(3):158-66.

[38] Ramachandran VS, Rogers Ramachandran D, Cobb S. Touching the phantom limb. Nature 1995;377(6549):489-90.

[39] Brodie EE, Whyte A, Waller B. Increased motor control of a phantom leg in humans results from the visual feedback of a virtual leg. Neurosci Lett 2003;341(2):167-9.

[40] Hunter JP, Katz J, Davis KD. The effect of tactile and visual sensory inputs on phantom limb awareness. Brain 2003;126(Pt 3):579-89.

[41] Brodie EE, Whyte A, Niven CA. Analgesia through the looking-glass? A randomized controlled trial investigating the effect of viewing a 'virtual' limb upon phantom limb pain, sensation and movement. Eur J Pain 2007;11(4):428-36.

[42] Chan BL, Witt R, Charrow AP, Magee A, Howard R, Pasquina PF, et al. Mirror therapy for phantom limb pain. N Engl J Med 2007;357(21):2206-7.

[43] Rock I, Victor J. Vision and Touch: An Experimentally Created Conflict between the Two Senses. Science 1964;143:594-6.

[44] Halligan PW, Hunt M, Marshall JC, Wade DT. When seeing is feeling; acquired synaesthesia or phantom touch? Neurocase 1996;2:21-29.

[45] Diers M, Christmann C, Koeppe C, Ruf M, Flor H. Mirrored, imagined and executed movements differentially activate sensorimotor cortex in amputees with and without phantom limb pain. Pain 2010;149(2):296-304.

[46] Moseley GL, Gallace A, Spence C. Is mirror therapy all it is cracked up to be? Current evidence and future directions. Pain 2008;138(1):7-10.

[47] Lotze M, Montoya P, Erb M, Hülsemann E, Flor H, Klose U, et al. Activation of cortical and cerebellar motor areas during executed and imagined hand movements: an fMRI study. Journal of Cognitive Neuroscience 1999;11(5):491-501.

[48] Ersland L, Rosén G, Lundervold A, Smievoll AI, Tillung T, Hugdahl S, et al. Phantom limb imaginary fingertapping causes primary motor cortex activation: an fMRI study. Neuro Report 1996;8(1):207-210.

[49] Roux FE, Lotterie JA, Cassol E, Lazorthes Y, Sol JC, Berry I. Cortical areas involved in virtual movement of phantom limbs: comparison with normal subjects. Neurosurgery 2003;53(6):1342-53.

[50] Roux FE, Ibarrola D, Lazorthes Y, Berry I. Virtual movements activate primary sensorimotor areas in amputees: report of three cases. Neurosurgery 2001;49(3):736-42.

[51] Mercier C, Reilly KT, Vargas CD, Aballea A, Sirigu A. Mapping phantom movement representations in the motor cortex of amputees. Brain 2006;129(Pt 8):2202-10.

[52] Giraux P, Sirigu A. Illusory movements of the paralyzed limb restore motor cortex activity. Neuroimage 2003;20 Suppl 1:S107-11.

Sensorimotor training and its implication for cortical reorganization   89

[53] MacIver K, Lloyd DM, Kelly S, Roberts N, Nurmikko T. Phantom limb pain, cortical reorganization and the therapeutic effect of mental imagery. Brain 2008;131(Pt 8):2181-91.

[54] Moseley GL. Graded motor imagery is effective for long-standing complex regional pain syndrome: a randomised controlled trial. Pain 2004;108(1-2):192-8.

[55] Moseley GL. Is successful rehabilitation of complex regional pain syndrome due to sustained attention to the affected limb? A randomised clinical trial. Pain 2005;114(1-2):54-61.

[56] Moseley GL. Graded motor imagery for pathologic pain: a randomized controlled trial. Neurology 2006;67(12):2129-34.

[57] McCabe CS, Haigh RC, Ring EF, Halligan PW, Wall PD, Blake DR. A controlled pilot study of the utility of mirror visual feedback in the treatment of complex regional pain syndrome (type 1). Rheumatology (Oxford) 2003;42(1):97-101.

[58] Gieteling EW, van Rijn MA, de Jong BM, Hoogduin JM, Renken R, van Hilten JJ, et al. Cerebral activation during motor imagery in complex regional pain syndrome type 1 with dystonia. Pain 2008;134(3):302-9.

[59] Pleger B, Janssen F, Schwenkreis P, Volker B, Maier C, Tegenthoff M. Repetitive transcranial magnetic stimulation of the motor cortex attenuates pain perception in complex regional pain syndrome type I. Neurosci Lett 2004;356(2):87-90.

[60] Ramachandran VS, Seckel EL. Using mirror visual feedback and virtual reality to treat fibromyalgia. Med Hypotheses 2010;in press.

[61] Moseley GL. I can't find it! Distorted body image and tactile dysfunction in patients with chronic back pain. Pain 2008;140(1):239-43.

[62] Bray H, Moseley GL. Disrupted working body schema of the trunk in people with back pain. Br J Sports Med 2010;in press.

[63] Thieme K, Flor H, Turk DC. Psychological pain treatment in fibromyalgia syndrome: efficacy of operant behavioural and cognitive behavioural treatments. Arthritis Res Ther 2006;8(4):R121.

[64] Thieme K, Gromnica-Ihle E, Flor H. Operant behavioral treatment of fibromyalgia: a controlled study. Arthritis Rheum 2003;49(3):314-20.

[65] Cole J. Virtual and augmented reality, phantom experience and prosthetics. In: Gallagher P, Desmond DM, MacLachlan M, editors. Neuroprostheses. London: Springer; 2007. p. 141-153.

[66] Desmond DM, O'Neill K, De Paor A, McDarby G, MacLachlan M. Augmenting the Reality of Phantom Limbs: Three Case Studies Using an Augmented Mirror Box Procedure. J Prosthet Orthot. 2006;18(3):74–79.

[67] Murray CD, Patchick E, Pettifer S, Caillette F, Howard T. Immersive virtual reality as a rehabilitative technology for phantom limb experience: a protocol. Cyberpsychol Behav 2006;9(2):167-70.

[68] Murray CD, Patchick EL, Caillette F, Howard T, Pettifer S. Can immersive virtual reality reduce phantom limb pain? Stud Health Technol Inform 2006;119:407-12.

[69] Murray CD, Pettifer S, Howard T, Patchick EL, Caillette F, Kulkarni J, et al. The treatment of phantom limb pain using immersive virtual reality: three case studies. Disabil Rehabil 2007;29(18):1465-9.

[70] Cole J, Crowle S, Austwick G, Slater DH. Exploratory findings with virtual reality for phantom limb pain; from stump motion to agency and analgesia. Disabil Rehabil 2009;31(10):846-54.

[71] Ehrsson HH, Rosen B, Stockselius A, Ragno C, Kohler P, Lundborg G. Upper limb amputees can be induced to experience a rubber hand as their own. Brain 2008;131(Pt 12):3443-52.

[72] Rossini PM, Micera S, Benvenuto A, Carpaneto J, Cavallo G, Citi L, et al. Double nerve intraneural interface implant on a human amputee for robotic hand control. Clin Neurophysiol 2010;121(5):777-83.

[73] Johnson S, Summers J, Pridmore S. Changes to somatosensory detection and pain thresholds following high frequency repetitive TMS of the motor cortex in individuals suffering from chronic pain. Pain 2006;123(1-2):187-92.

[74] Sampson SM, Rome JD, Rummans TA. Slow-frequency rTMS reduces fibromyalgia pain. Pain Med 2006;7(2):115-8.

[75] Fregni F, Gimenes R, Valle AC, Ferreira MJ, Rocha RR, Natalle L, et al. A randomized, sham-controlled, proof of principle study of transcranial direct current stimulation for the treatment of pain in fibromyalgia. Arthritis Rheum 2006;54(12):3988-98.

[76] Antal A, Terney D, Kuhnl S, Paulus W. Anodal transcranial direct current stimulation of the motor cortex ameliorates chronic pain and reduces short intracortical inhibition. J Pain Symptom Manage;39(5):890-903.

[77] Fregni F, Freedman S, Pascual-Leone A. Recent advances in the treatment of chronic pain with non-invasive brain stimulation techniques. Lancet Neurol 2007;6(2):188-91.

[78] Williams JA, Imamura M, Fregni F. Updates on the use of non-invasive brain stimulation in physical and rehabilitation medicine. J Rehabil Med 2009;41(5):305-11.

Chapter VI

The role of mental imagery in chronic deafferentation pain and its effect on cortical reorganization

Kate MacIver, RGN, MSC, Paul Sacco, PhD and Turo Nurmikko, MD, PhD*

Pain Research Institute, University of Liverpool,
Clinical Sciences Centre, Liverpool, UK

Abstract

The aim of this chapter is to review mental imagery, its effect on cortical plasticity and its role in the management of chronic pain, with particular reference to chronic deafferentation pain. Normal mechanisms of neuroplasticity are outlined, including changes in somatotopic representation at cortical level. Neuroplasticity in response to damage to the central and peripheral nervous systems is also discussed, and the relationship between maladaptive cortical reorganization and pain. The resistance of many deafferentation pain syndromes to standard

---

* Correspondence: Kate MacIver, RGN MSC, Faculty of Health and Life Sciences, University of Liverpool, Clinical Sciences Centre, Lower Lane, Liverpool, L9 7AL, United Kingdom. E-mail: kmaciver@liv.ac.uk

pharmacotherapy has led to researchers to seek alternative methods of management, and much work has been done to study ways of reducing the maladaptive cortical reorganization and malfunction linked to nervous system injury and pain. Mental imagery in various forms has been used with varying degrees of success, and the main focus of this paper is to review the literature relating to these therapies. We can conclude that mental imagery shows promise as a means of alleviating these distressing conditions.

Introduction

Advances in our understanding of the function of the brain have led to major discoveries of the mechanisms that generate and maintain chronic pain. Pain signals reaching the brain are processed through an extensive neural network connecting several areas associated with somatosensation and emotion, in conjunction with areas that prepare for motor action. Disease and injury, especially affecting the peripheral or central nervous systems, lead to major neuroplastic changes throughout the brain and can be reliably measured using functional brain imaging. Early results suggest that not only are such changes critical for the development of pain but they can also be modulated by various methods. In this review we will concentrate on the role of motor imagery for the control of chronic pain and discuss the rationale behind this approach.

Mechanisms of neuroplasticity

Neuroplasticity refers to the ability of the central nervous system to adapt in response to physiological demand, environmental pressures or familiarity with a given task (1). Cortical plasticity is defined as the preferential allocation of cortical space to those peripheral areas proportionately most in use (2). Depending on the nature of the demand, dynamic neuronal plasticity may be transient and rapidly responsive, dependent upon presynaptic firing rate and neurotransmitter release (3) and just as rapidly return to its previous state when the challenge diminishes. In contrast, long-term plasticity is slower, relying on different mechanisms such as dendritic growth and arborisation (4). This ability to undergo adaptation is intrinsic in all components of the central nervous system at a cellular, biochemical, structural and functional level (1), from spinal cord to brain (5).

The immature brain responds to alterations in sensory input by changing its structural make-up (6). Neuronal pathways are mapped out under genetic blueprints and then the circuits are strengthened, maintained and adjusted by the neuronal activity itself. In contrast, the adult brain is less flexible, albeit still capable of responding to sensory challenges by forming new neuronal connections. Adaptive and maladaptive neuroplasticity occurs most commonly in response to a change in sensory input whether it is an increase, a reduction or a cessation of afferent information (7).

Central nervous system somatotopic representation of the body

The cortical and sub-cortical systems contain two distinct neural maps – one for the recognition and processing of sensory input (sensory homunculus), and the other one for the delivery of motor commands (motor homunculus) (8). Sensory and motor maps have an orderly, somatotopic arrangement of neural connections to represent each area of the body, an arrangement first localized along the central sulci in both hemispheres, using electrical stimulation during brain surgery for epilepsy (see Figure 1) (9).

These primary motor (M1) and sensory (S1) cortical areas are the final, macroscopic areas of plasticity, however recent research has shown, and is focusing on, somatotopic organisation at all levels of the brain, from brainstem to cortex (10). Somatotopic reorganization generally occurs in cortical and subcortical areas, but changes in cortical somatotopy may occur regardless of subcortical input (11). Sensory maps are widespread throughout the cortex and other areas of the brain and these functional maps are able to respond rapidly to changes in efferent input, as all cortical neurons possess an intrinsic excitability. Somatosensory maps develop at an early stage in embryonic development, yet retain their capacity to respond and change in the face of external influences and behaviours (12). Other sensory modalities, such as hearing and some aspects of vision are time-sensitive, and their ability to change is lost in adulthood (5), hence damage to vision or hearing does not improve with time.

In normal life, cortical reorganization is an adaptive process which is essential for our everyday functioning. One of the most important elements of plastic adaptation is the fact that the nervous system is able to revert back to pre-challenge circuits once the challenge has either been met or dissipated.

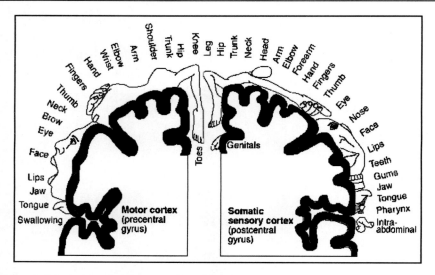

Figure 1. Diagrammatic representation of primary motor and sensory homunculi.

However cortical reorganization can become maladaptive, with or without injury or disease of the nervous system. For example in the case of professional, classical musicians, who need to perform stereotypical, repetitive movements of the hands and/or mouth for several hours per day, there is a 1% incidence of dystonia (13). Musician's dystonia has been correlated with an over-representation of the hand cortical motor map and both are reduced by proprioceptive retraining and changes to musical practice (14).

When the nervous system is damaged, for example during amputation or spinal cord injury, the patterns of reorganization may be different. Jones (12) reviewed the published data from experimental studies on the different neuroplastic responses to loss of sensory input and conversely increased sensory input resulting from intensive practice of a motor task. He concluded that sensory loss due to amputation results in the invasion of the deafferented cortical representational map by adjacent areas on the homunculus. In contrast, extraordinary stimulation of a body part such as the digits will result in an enlargement in the cortical representational map of that body part. In adaptive plasticity, the increased neuronal activation remains confined to the normal representation in the cortices, whereas following trauma to the nervous system (amputation or spinal injury) the increased neural activity occurs in adjacent areas. The latter neuroplastic change may in some cases have a disadvantageous effect and be maladaptive, for example in phantom pain following amputation of a limb (15). In some situations this "deprivation-dependent" plasticity may have the additional adaptive effect of allowing the individual to harness the deafferented brain cells to promote recovery of function, such as is seen after stroke (12).

Cortical reorganization and chronic pain

It is now well documented that both sensory and motor cortical reorganization occurs as a result of amputation and is more extensive in those who suffer from phantom limb pain (PLP) (15,16). It has also been shown to occur in conjunction with other pain conditions such as complex regional pain syndrome (measured by functional Magnetic Resonance Imaging (fMRI) (17) and fibromyalgia (measured by Transcranial Magnetic Stimulation; TMS;18). In particular it is the pain syndromes associated with deafferentation causing sensory loss which are most obviously associated with cortical reorganization, and which are arguably most susceptible to manipulation.

So, in the case of maladaptive cortical reorganization aligned with deafferentation pain syndromes, is it possible to manipulate maladaptive cortical reorganization, and if so will this produce pain relief? Many of these pain conditions do not respond well to standard pharmacological therapy and there is a need for good clinical management. It is possible to modulate the excitability of the motor cortex using techniques such as motor cortex stimulation (MCS), TMS or transcranial direct current stimulation (tDCS), and these techniques have been used to treat neuropathic pain (19), although their mode of action remains unclear. There is however another, simpler method of modifying cortical activity – mental imagery.

Mental imagery

Kosslyn and colleagues (20) argue that mental imagery is a skill used in everyday life. Mental practice enables us to rehearse and then remember a sequence of tasks or a list, to recall information or to improve motor skills such as a sequence of dance steps. Most mental images are generated from a store of past experience served up with a dose of imagination. Plato believed that memory was called up from a store of images etched onto the brain, like words on a wax tablet and other psychological theories in later times set much store by mental images or the internalized working of the mind (20). The popularity of behavioural theories of psychology saw a decline in interest in mental imagery, but the emergence of cognitive psychology in the 1970's led to a resurgence of interest in the process of mental imagery and its therapeutic value.

Mental imagery can be defined as percepts or sensations generated internally by the brain, a mental representation of an actual sensation or movement, for example seeing pictures in "the mind's eye," hearing voices or imagining movement of the fingers (21). So accurate is this representation that it follows the rules of Fitts' Law (22) which states that the speed of a movement may be sacrificed in order to ensure its accuracy, and vice versa – this is still the case if a movement is imagined rather than actually performed (23). Sirigu and colleagues also established that imagined movement is constrained by the capacity of the body to undertake the actual movement, such that, when physical impairment (in this case cerebral stroke) inhibited the performance of an action, then the motor imagery was perceived to be likewise impaired. Early physiological studies showed that motor imagery resulted in increased excitability of the corticospinal pathways and, if the motor imagery was perceived to be strenuous, increased pulse and respiratory rates. This provided indirect support for the idea that imagined movements shared the same cortical pathways as the executed motor task (24).

Further evidence for the congruence of the neural pathways of imagined and executed movements have come from more recent TMS studies. Firstly changes in excitability of the corticospinal pathways during imagined movements are highly specific, such that changes can be focused to individual finger movements. This is despite the highly interconnected nature of the representation of the intrinsic hand muscles in the motor cortex (25). Furthermore Hashimoto and Rothwell (26) showed that when subjects imagined performing continuous wrist flexion and extension movements, the TMS responses of the wrist flexor muscles were larger during the flexion phase of the imagined movement. Thus the imagined movements showed the same phasic changes in excitability found during actual movement. Interestingly, they also found that the wrist extensor responses were smaller during imagined flexion compared to the resting state. This inhibitory effect of motor imagery on corticomotor excitability has been confirmed by Sohn and colleagues (27) who showed that excitability of cortico-motor pathways to the hand can be reduced using "negative" motor imagery. In addition, mental imagery of a specific task can improve the executed performance of that task (see for example, 28; 29; 30) but only if the executed task has been previously performed or attempted, and usually in concert with active practice.

Visual, auditory and kinaesthetic imagery have been shown to activate the same cortical areas as actual vision, hearing and movement (24). This review of the literature will focus on motor imagery which is the most commonly used as a clinical intervention for chronic pain.

Cerebral mechanisms of motor imagery and motor performance

The links between actual and imagined performance of a motor task can be traced to the cerebral mechanisms responsible (30). An important element of this is efference copy which occurs in both the sensory and motor systems, although much of the earlier research studied the visual systems (31). To overcome the inevitable delay which would occur between a movement and the sensory confirmation that the movement has been executed there is a forward sensory model, or memory store of the predictable sensations, which is activated at the same time as the motor cortical command and is known as the efference copy – i.e. a downstream activation predicting the consequences of the motor action (32). Such a feedforward model allows us to make automatic movements such as gait adjustment without a constant barrage of sensory feedback. Christensen and colleagues used ischaemic nerve block to eradicate proprioceptive feedback and then used fMRI and connectivity analysis to measure areas of the brain responsible for the efference copy of sensory signals during movement of an anaesthetized limb. The largest increase in activity during nerve block occurred in the ventral premotor and primary sensory cortices, with significant connectivity between the two. The authors conclude that descending modulation of primary sensory cortices by premotor cortex is the source of predictive efference copy. These results are in agreement with the findings of Voss et al (33) who used TMS to determine changes to sensory perception in moving and resting fingers. When primary motor cortex output was blocked by TMS there was a concomitant sensory attenuation, which the authors conclude was due to activity in the motor preparation areas of the brain, i.e. premotor cortex. So, premotor cortex, responsible for preparation and planning of motor activity also ensures the smooth running of bodily movement by damping down sensory feedback when necessary by using a pre-prepared (or efference) copy. This efference copy is important for the generation of motor imagery (21) and brain imaging studies of motor imagery consistently report activation in premotor and supplementary motor areas (SMA) (30).

Imaging and imagining

Brain imaging studies of the mechanisms and consequences of motor imagery have been undertaken in both healthy volunteers and clinical groups. Results of studies of activation during motor imagery can be compared with activation in response to executed movement, using fMRI to map precisely the activation of somatotopic representations in primary motor and sensory cortices in response to the execution of simple tasks (34,35). Using Magnetoencephalography (MEG) and fMRI Lotze and colleagues (36) were able to show that executed and imagined movement of the hand activated ipsilateral cerebellum and contralateral primary motor cortex (M1). Although previous studies using fMRI had also shown M1 activation during imagined movement (37,38), these researchers did not control for unobserved minute executed movements during the experiment, a confounding factor in many studies of motor imagery when electromyelography (EMG) is not used to measure any unwanted executed movement (30). An alternative to EMG is to observe the individual closely during imagery to eliminate the possibility of inadvertent executed movement (39). Ehrsson and colleagues (40) used fMRI to measure responses to imagined movement of the fingers, toes and tongue with resultant activation in contralateral, somatotopically correct motor cortex (i.e. hand area for imagined hand movement and so on) but also activation in SMA and premotor areas. In a small study of 6 sportsmen, Ogiso and colleagues (41) used MEG to measure brain activation in response to imagining hurdling as a means of improving actual performance, and found activation not only in SMA and premotor areas but also in precuneus. The precuneus is the posteromedial area of the parietal lobe, and plays a pivotal role in highly connective tasks such as visuo-spatial imagery and episodic memory tasks (42). Other studies of imagery which have not shown precuneus activation have been those of simple, internal imaginary tasks such as finger movement, as opposed to the complex spatial tasks used in the study by Ogiso and colleagues (41). Thus it seems that premotor cortical areas are important for the generation of internal imagined tasks such as movement of body parts, with precuneus having an additional role when the imagined tasks involve an external view of the self performing a complex task, with or without props.

Imagery in clinical populations

The converging evidence that motor imagery can activate the same areas of the brain as executed movement has led to studies in clinical populations where motor imagery has been utilised as a potential therapeutic intervention. These interventions focus on neurorehabilitation, for example after stroke, or management of deafferentation pain.

Can brain plasticity be manipulated to improve function during rehabilitation after stroke? Converging evidence suggests that this is the case. Sirigu and colleagues (23) showed that following stroke, people retain an ability to imagine movement of the paraparetic limb by accessing the cerebral motor pathways. Cramer and Crafton (43) used fMRI to determine that, although motor somatotopy was for the most part intact after stroke, there was a medial shift of the face representation into the deafferented hand area. Constraint therapy, where the unaffected arm is immobilized for several hours per day to force the person to use the affected arm for simple activities of daily living, has been shown to result in functional improvement as the brain adapts by expanding connectivity into undamaged areas, thus capitalizing on neuroplasticity (44,45). Training in motor imagery of the affected limbs also produces an improvement in functional recovery. In a review of five fMRI studies, Sharma and colleagues highlighted a functional improvement, with activation in response to motor imagery in SMA, premotor cortex and cerebellum – the predictive motor pathway. In the case of motor imagery, they concluded that those most likely to benefit from motor imagery were those without damage to the primary motor or parietal areas, i.e. those with subcortical stroke, and who have also retained some residual function of the affected limb.

The therapeutic use of mental imagery for the management of chronic, deafferentation pain

The fact that motor imagery can activate the same cerebral motor circuits as executed movement; that this is the case in both healthy and clinical populations and that mental imagery is easy to learn and to practice has meant that pain clinicians have been tempted to study the use of this technique in pain management, particularly in the area of chronic deafferentation pain. One reason for this is the lack of definitive pharmacological or surgical answers to this resistant clinical problem (46). In particular work has been done with people with phantom limb pain, complex regional pain syndrome (CRPS) and deafferentation pain following spinal cord injury and these studies will be discussed here.

Perhaps the first imagery technique to be used for deafferentation pain is the mirror box, developed by Ramachandran (47). The missing sensory afferent feedback is provided by a mirror reflection of the intact hand, which when moved gives the illusion of additional movement of the missing or painful hand, and has been used with mixed success for PLP and CRPS (48). Moseley (49) had better results using a graded motor imagery programme in a group of patients with either PLP or CRPS. In this randomised trial participants in the active treatment group were given a combination of limb laterality recognition (using photographs of hands in various positions), graded motor imagery (imagining movement of the missing or painful hand) and mirror box therapy over a six week training period, compared to a group receiving standard physiotherapy. The active treatment was effective in reducing both the pain and disability of CRPS and PLP.

Evidence from neurophysiological, neuroanatomic and clinical studies of amputation of a limb confirms neuroplastic changes in somatosensory and motor cortices (50). There is a shift of activation from neighbouring somatotopic representations towards deafferented areas in both motor (51) and sensory maps (52) and these shifts are significantly correlated with the intensity of phantom limb pain (16). This cortical reorganization following limb amputation has been shown to reduce following training in mental imagery (imagining normal sensation and purposeful movement in the missing limb) with a concomitant reduction in phantom limb pain (53).

In our study of the therapeutic effect of mental imagery on PLP related to upper limb amputation, we used a combination of a body scan (based on mindfulness meditation) and motor and sensory imagery (53). Mindfulness meditation has its roots in Buddhism, is commonly used in the west without the connotations of religion or culture and has been adapted for use in various modes of clinical practice (54). The main focus of the body scan is to concentrate attention on internally generated experiences, including the breath, sensations from consecutive areas of the body, thoughts, feelings and environmental stimuli (55). This practice contributes to a state of "mindfulness" which is the ability to focus on each immediate moment with curiosity and acceptance, but without judgment or emotional response (56). Within the context of this relaxing exercise, participants were then taught to incorporate the missing limb into to the body schema by imagining the presence of normal sensations such as the touch of a sleeve or pressure from the arm of a chair. Following this participants were encouraged to imagine comfortable and thorough movement of the phantom limb, such that they could "stretch away the pain" and then finally to imagine the limb coming to rest in a comfortable position. The full therapy session lasted approximately 40 minutes, with the movement component lasting about 5 minutes. Participants were seen individually once a week for 6 weeks and given a CD of the body scan and imagined movement and encouraged to practice daily at home. They were also taught a short form of the exercise, lasting about 10 minutes so that they could imagine movement and sensation in the missing limb without needing the CD, and were encouraged to practice the movement element of the therapy several times per day. The rationale behind the format of the therapy was to repeatedly challenge the displaced cortical activity with sensation and movement perceived to be coming from the phantom limb, and that this would need to be done regularly throughout the day to stimulate the abnormal cerebral activity patterns. 9 of the 13 participants in this pilot study gained > 50% pain relief by the end of the therapy. Functional brain imaging showed a reduction in cortical reorganization demonstrated by lip purse (as 16) from face area to hand area (see Figure 2).

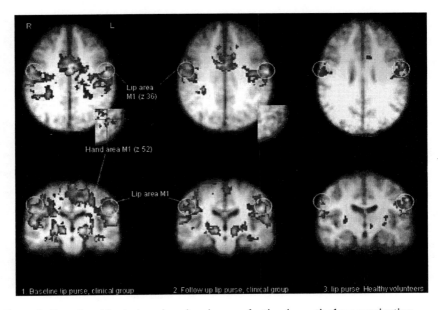

Figure 2. Functional brain imaging showing a reduction in cortical reorganization.

In the case of spinal cord injury, mental imagery has also been shown to activate primary and secondary motor pathways, and indeed to exceed the activation in response to motor imagery in healthy controls (57) which Alkhadi suggests is due to a lack of inhibitory sensory feedback. Cramer et al (39) hypothesized that, because mental imagery activates the same brain areas as executed movement, it could be utilized to change abnormal cerebral reorganization patterns despite the lack of normal bodily function.

They emphasized the importance of this in the light of new research into repair of the damaged spinal cord and the need to demonstrate functional connections from spinal cord to brain.

This group used an external form of motor imagery whereby participants learned to imagine plantarflexion of the right foot to crush a variety of computer-generated objects. After training they showed an increase in activation in contralateral thalamus, putamen and M1, but did not discuss activation in precuneus, which might be expected given the external nature of the imagery.

A limitation of this study is the small study population (10 in each group of healthy controls and spinal injured) the drop out of three controls and the loss of five fMRI data sets in the SCI groups because of excessive head motion.

Gustin and colleagues (58) studied 11 people with complete thoracic SCI and below level neuropathic pain and 19 healthy controls, using fMRI to measure activation in response to imagined movement of the toes, with similar results to Alkhadi and colleagues (57), in that there was activation in contralateral primary motor cortex, SMA and ipsilateral cerebellum. In this study, the mental imagery exercise consisted of training over a 7-day period to imagine pressing a car accelerator with the right paralyzed foot, and in several of the patients this either evoked new pain or provoked existing below level pain, the authors arguing that the imaginary movement activated the pain matrix, in particular the insula and anterior cingulate cortices.

The motor imagery training was carried out for one week prior to fMRI scanning, with the intention that the participants would be competent in motor imagery during the scanning procedure. It was not intended as a therapeutic intervention for pain relief.

Combining mental imagery with other forms of therapy

The ease of mental imagery and its internal derivation make the technique highly suitable for use in combination with other forms of modulation in the treatment of chronic neuropathic pain. Such an approach has recently been described by Soler and colleagues (59) who studied the effects of tDCS, virtual walking illusion imagery and combined tDCS / imagery in a group of 40 subjects with neuropathic pain following SCI. Whilst tDCS therapy and motor imagery in isolation provided significant amelioration of pain symptoms, the group receiving the combined therapy had more effective and long lasting pain relief. Such findings indicate the promise of motor imagery as an adjuvant therapy and more studies of this nature are clearly indicated.

In conclusion, recent brain imaging studies in patients show that following injury the central nervous system undergoes major neuroplastic changes, some of which are maladaptive and contribute to the development and maintenance of chronic pain. Maladaptive cortical reorganization can be reduced my motor imagery, and early results suggest it also results in an improvement in pain. Motor imagery therefore appears to be a promising tool in the management of chronic pain, especially in conditions which are traditionally seen to be refractory to conventional treatment. Whether individual patients with defined deafferentation pain syndromes will benefit best from internally generated imagery or externally generated imagery (with or without visual aids such as a mirror box or computer generated images) and perhaps enhanced by direct stimulation of the cortex using TMS or tDCS are questions for future studies.

References

[1] Pascual-Leone A, Amedi A, Fregni F, Merabet LB. The Plastic Human Cortex. Annu Rev Neuroscience 2005;28:377-401.

[2] Buonomano DV, Merzenich M. Cortical plasticity: from synapse to maps. Annu Rev Neuroscience 1998;21:149-86.

[3] Engelman HS, MacDermott. A. Presynaptic ionotropic receptors and control of transmitter release. Nat Rev Neurosci 2004;5:135-45.

[4] Kelly C, Garavan H. Human neuroimaging of brain changes associated with practice. Cereb Cortex 2005;15:1089-102.

[5] Wolpaw JR, Tennissen. A. Activity-dependent spinal cord plasticity in health and disease. Annu Rev Neuroscience 2001;24:807-43.

[6] Knott G, Holtmaat A. Denriditic spine plasticity - current understanding from in vivo studies. Brain Res Rev 2008;58:282-9.

[7] Hickmott PW, Merzenich MM. Local circuit properties underlying cortical reorganization. J Neurophysiol 2002;88:1288-301.

[8] Amaral DG. The functional organisation of perception and movement. In: Kandel ER, Schwartz JH, Jessell TM eds., Principles of neural science, 4th ed. New York: McGraw-Hill, 2000:337-48.

[9] Penfield W, Boldrey E. Somatic motor and sensory representation in the cerebral cortex of man as studied by electrical stimulation. Brain 1937;60:389-443.

[10] Romanelli P, Esposito V, Schaal DW, Heit G. Somatotopy of the basal ganglia: experimental and clinical evidence for segregated sensorimotor channels. Brain Res Rev 2005;48:112-28.

[11] Hickmott PW. Changes in intrinsic properties of pyramidal neurons in adult rat S1 during cortical reorganization. J Neurophysiol 2005;94:501-11.

[12] Jones EG. Cortical and subcortical contributions to activity-dependent plasticity in the primate somatosensory cortex. Annu Rev Neurosci 2000;23:1-37.

[13] Altenmuller E, Jabusch H.-C. Focal dystonia in musicians: phenomenology, pathophysiology and triggering factors. Eur J Neurol 2010;17(Suppl):31-6.

[14] Rosenkratz K, Butler K, Williamon A, Rothwell JC. Regaining motor control in musician's dystonia by restoring sensorimotor organisation. J Neurosci 2009;29:14627-36.

[15] Flor H, Elbert T, Knecht S, Wienbruch C, Pantev C, Birbaumer N, Larbig W, Taub E. Phantom-limb pain as a correlate of cortical reorganization following arm amputation. Nature 1995;375:482-4.

[16] Lotze M, Flor H, Grodd W, Larbig W, Birbaumer N. Phantom movements and pain: an fMRI study in upper limb amputees. Brain 2001;124:2268-77.

[17] Seifert F, Maihofner C. Central mechanisms of neuropathic pain: findings from functional imaging studies. Cell Mol Life Sci 2009;66:375-90.

[18] Mhalla A, de Andrade BC, Baudic S, Perrot S, Bouhasssira D. Alteration of cortical excitability in patients with fibromyalgia. Pain 2009;149:495-500.

[19] Lefaucher JP. Methods of therapeutic cortical stimulation. Neurophysiol Clin 2009;39:1-14.

[20] Kosslyn SM, Behrmann M, Jeannerod M. The cognitive neuroscience of mental imagery. Neuropsychologia 1995;33:1335-44.

[21] Moulton ST, Kosslyn SM. Imagining predictions: mental imagery as mental emulation. Phil Trans R Soc Lond 2009;364:1273-80.

[22] Fitts P. The information capacity of the human motor system in controlling the amplitude of movement. J Exp Psychol 1954;47:381-91.

[23] Sirugu A, Duhamel J-R, Cohen L, Pillon B, Dubois B, Aqid Y. The mental representation of hand movements after parietal damage. Science 1996;173:1564-68.

[24] Annett J. Motor imagery: perception or action? Neuropsychologia 1995;33:1395-1417.

[25] Rossini PM, Rossi S, Pasqualetti P, Tecchio F. Corticospinal excitability modulation to hand muscles during movement imagery. Cereb Cortex 1999;9:161-7.

[26] Hashimoto R, Rothwell JC. Dynamic changes in corticospinal excitability during motor imagery. Exp Brain Res 1999;125:75-81.

[27] Sohn YH, Dang N, Hallett M. Suppression of corticospinal excitability during negative motor imagery. J Neurophysiol 2003;90:2303-9.

[28] Gentili R, Papaxanthis C, Pozzo T. Improvement and generalization of arm motor performance through motor imagery practice. Neuroscience 2006;137:761-72.

[29] Karni A, Meyer G, Rey-Hippolito C, Jezzard P, Adams MM, Turner R, Ungerleider LG. The acquisition of skilled motor performance: fast and slow experience-driven changes in primary motor cortex. Proc Natl Acad Sci USA 1998;95:861-8.

[30] Lotze M, Halsband U. Motor imagery. J Physiol (Lond) 2006;99:386-95.

[31] Bridgeman B. A review of the role of efference copy in sensory and oculomotor control systems. Ann Biomed Engineering 1995;23:409-22.

[32] Christensen MS, Lundbye-Jensen J, Geersten SS, Petersen TH, Paulson OB, Nielsen JB. Premotor cortex modulates somatosensory cortex during voluntary movements without proprioceptive feedback. Nat Neurosci 2007;10:417-9.

[33] Voss M, Ingram JN. Sensorimotor attenuation by central motor command signals in the absence of movement. Nat Neurosci 2006;9:6-27.

[34] Yousry TA, Schmid H, Alkhadi H, Schmidt D, Peraud A, Buettner A et al. Localisation of motor hand area to a knob on the precentral gyrus. A new landmark. Brain 1997;120:141-57.

[35] Stippich C, Ochmann H, Satror K. Somatotopic mapping of the human primary sensorimotor cortex during motor imagery and execution during functional magentic resonance imaging. Neurosci Lett 2002:331:50-4.

[36] Lotze M, Montoya P, Erb M, Hulsmann E, Flor H, Klose U, Birbaumer N, Grodd W. Activation of cortical and cerebellar motor areas during executed and imagined hand movements: an fMRI study. J Cogn Neurosci 1999;11:491-501.

[37] Sabbah P, Simmond G, Levrier O, Habbib M, Traboud V, Murayama N, Matzoya BM, Briant JF, Raybaud C, Salomon G. Functional magnetic resonance imaging at 1.5T during sensory, motor and cognitive tasks. Eur Neurol 1995;35:131-6.

[38] Porro CA, Cettolo V, Francescatoraldi P. Primary motor and sensory cortex activation during motor performance and motor imagery: a functional magnetic resonance imaging study. J Neurosci 1996;16:7688-98.

[39] Cramer SC, Orr ELR, Cohen MJ, Lacourse MG. Effects of motor imagery training after complete spinal cord injury. Exp Brain Res 2007;177:233-242.

[40] Ehrsson HH, Geyer S, Naito E. Imagery of voluntary movement of fingers, toes and tongue activates corresponding body-part-specific motor representations. J Neurophysiol 2003;90:3304-16.

[41] Ogiso T, Kobayashi K, Sugishita M. The precuneus in mental imagery: a magnetoencephalographic study. Neuroreport 2000;11:1345-9.

[42] Cavanna AE, Trimble R. The precuneus: a review of its functional anatomy and behvaioural correlates. Brain 2006;129:564-83.

[43] Cramer SC, Crafton K. Somatotopy and movement representation sites following cortical stroke. Exp Brain Research 2006;168:25-32.

[44] Sharma N, Pomeroy VM, Baron J-C. Motor imagery: a backdoor to the motor system after stroke? Stroke 2006;37:1941-52.

[45] Liepert J, Bauder H, Miltner WHR, Taub E, Weiller C. Treatment-induced cortical reorganization after stroke in humans. Stroke 2000;31:1210-6.

[46] Birklein F, Maihofner C. Use your imagination: training the brain and not the body to improve chronic pain and restore function. Neurology 2006;67:2115-6.

[47] Ramachandran VS, Rogers-Ramachandran D. Synaesthesia in phantom limbs induced with mirrors. Proc R Soc Lond B Biol Sci 1996;263:377-86.

[48] Moseley GL, Gallace A, Spence C. Is mirror therapy all it's cracked up to be? Current evidence and future directions. Pain 2008;138:7-10.

[49] Moseley GL. Graded motor imagery for pathologic pain: a randomised controlled trial. Neurology 2006;67:1-6.

[50] Flor H. Maladaptive plasticity, memory for pain and phantom limb pain: review and suggestions for new therapies. Expert Rev Neurother 2008;8:809-19.

[51] Chen R, Cohen LG, Hallett M. Nervous system reorganization following injury. Neuroscience 2002;111:761-73.

[52] Mackert B-M, Sappok T, Grusser S, Flor H, Curio G. The eloquence of silent cortex. Neuroreport 2003;14:409-12.

[53] MacIver K, Lloyd DM, Kelly S, Roberts N, Nurmikko T. Phantom limb pain, cortical reorganization and the therapeutic effects of mental imagery. Brain 2008;131:2181-91.

[54] Ospina MB, Bond K, Karkaneh M, Tjosvold L, Vandermeer B, Liang Y et al. Meditation practices for health - state of the research. Evidence Report / Technology Assessment 2007;155:AHRQ Publication No. 07-E010.

[55] Wahbeh H, Elsas S-M, Oken BS. Mind body interventions: applications in neurology. Neurology 2008;70:2321-8.

[56] Bishop SR. What do we really know about mindfulness meditation? Psychosom Med 2002;64:1-84.

[57] Alkhadi H, Brugger P, Boen H, Crelier G, Curt A, Hepp-Raymond M-C, Kollias SS. What disconnection tells us about motor imagery: evidence from paraplegic patients. Cereb Cortex 2005;15:131-40.

[58] Gustin SM, Wrigley P, Henderson LA, Siddall P. Brain circuitry underlying pain in response to imagined movement in people with spinal cord injury. Pain 2010;148:438-45.

[59] Soler MD, Kumru H, Pelayo R, Vidal J, Tormos JM, Navarro X et al. Effectiveness of transcranial direct current stimulation and visual illusion on neuropathic pain in spinal cord injury. Brain 2010;133:2565-77.

Chapter VII

Functional and structural cortical neuroplasticity in trigeminal neuropathic pain

*Marcos FH DosSantos, DDS, MSc and Alexandre F DaSilva, DDS, DMedSc**
Headache and Orofacial Pain Effort (HOPE),
Biologic and Materials Sciences,
University of Michigan, School of Dentistry,
Ann Arbor, Michigan, US

Abstract

Trigeminal neuropathic pain (TNP) is a chronic disorder with problematical prognosis. The fact that multiple therapeutic modalities provide modest relief for these patients raises the possibility that the cause for the chronicity of this debilitating disorder may also lie within the brain itself. Notably, recent reports stemming primarily from neuroimaging have indicated that the prolonged experience of pain and suffering in such patients may result in resistant changes in the cortical milieu. Hence, even if the original etiologic factor is removed or

---

* Correspondence: Alexandre F. DaSilva DDS, DMedSc, Director, Headache and Orofacial Pain Effort (H.O.P.E.) TM, Biologic and Materials Sciences, University of Michigan, School of Dentistry, 1011 N. University Ave., Room 1014A, Ann Arbor, MI 48109-107 United States. E-mail: adasilva@umich.edu

addressed, the pain is still unruly. Here, we describe how novel neuroimaging tools are elucidating the functional and structural neuroplasticity that occurs in the brain of TNP patients, and which cortical regions associated with pain perception are affected.

Introduction

According to the International Association for the Study of Pain (IASP), pain is defined as an experience associated with actual or potential tissue damage, which requires action to avoid extensive suffering and assists healing to ultimately reach homeostasis of the organism (1). Unfortunately, if not idiopathic, pain can persist beyond the removal of its cause, being spontaneous and/or evoked by a harmless non-noxious stimulus (allodynia). Neuropathic pain is the pain that develops after damage, disease or dysfunction of the peripheral or central nervous system (2). It is considered a clinical challenge whose current treatment options offer uncertain long-term benefits. The incidence is almost 1% per annum in the general population, and it tends to be more frequent with the increase of age and women are more affected than men (3). The mechanism is not totally elucidated, but it is largely assumed that both central and peripheral mechanisms play a role in neuropathic pain with the changes in the Central Nervous System (CNS) being, at least in part, determined by changes in the Peripheral Nervous System (PNS) (4, 5). Trigeminal neuropathic pain (TNP) disorders such as classical, atypical and postherpetic trigeminal neuralgias are examples of chronic neuropathic pain where our limited understanding of the pathophysiology adversely affects the development of less empirical and more effective treatment options. They are generally debilitating chronic conditions in which pain can be spontaneous or intensely evoked by harmless daily activities, such as eating, talking or by light touch to the facial skin (tactile allodynia). In TNP disorders, the normal sensory mechanism is altered leading to characteristic neuronal changes (5, 6).

Classical trigeminal neuralgia (classical-TN) on average affects elderly people with age at diagnosis of 67 years, and is rare below 40. It is usually described as a disorder with an incidence of 5.7 in women and 2.5 in men yearly per 100.000 persons, respectively in the US population (4, 7, 8). However, other studies reported different incidents in distinct populations (9-11). The pain is described as sharp or shooting. Paroxysmal pain is elicited mostly when the trigger point, frequently located in the oral or perioral region, is stimulated by light touch (evoked pain) (12). It is proposed that classical-TN is caused by compression and, consequently, demyelination of the trigeminal root by a blood vessel, usually the superior cerebellar artery loop, or tumors at the level of the cerebellopontine angle, specifically in the trigeminal root entry zone (REZ) (13). In contrast, atypical trigeminal neuralgia (atypical-TN) affects a large number of patients with a variety of pain patterns (14).Mild to severe pain in an area of trigeminal injury (trauma, surgery, tumor), is usually constant and exacerbated to a lesser degree by touch (spontaneous and evoked pain respectively) of the injury (15). It might result from injuries of the trigeminal nerve root but in this case the damage takes place in any point distal to the REZ (16-18). In addition, this condition can be sometimes associated to trauma or surgery in the orofacial region (19).

Another condition of TNP is postherpetic neuralgia (PHN). It is one of the most common conditions seen in the pain clinic (4). Although there is no standard definition for PHN, it can be defined as the neuropathic pain that follows a characteristic acute rash of Herpes Zoster or Shingles, a disease that predominantly affects the elderly population (20-23). PHN is associated with reactivation of the varicella zoster virus (VZV), mostly in the ophthalmic division of the trigeminal nerve (24-26). Most patients recover completely of herpes zoster after some months. However, in some of them, the pain persists after the rash healing, a condition defined as PHN (27, 28). It has been described that the incidence as well as the severity (measured by duration) of PHN is directly related to age. Also, it seems that there is no predilection for gender related to PHN (20, 24, 29-32). The symptoms are more constant atypical-like, for instance, deep burning pain associated with paroxysmal and lancinating pain. In addition, those patients commonly relate other sensory disturbances, such as allodynia, paresthesia, dysesthesia, hyperalgesia and itching (20, 33) (21). Notwithstanding some theories have been proposed to explain the mechanism of pain related to PHN its pathophysiology is not completely elucidated. Some recent studies have associated its occurrence to the density of epidermal innervation after Herpes Zoster infection (34).

The puzzling and sometimes overly simplistic current clinical and research view of the TNP disorders is primarily due to our limited understanding of their pathophysiology. Currently, there are no objective laboratory or pathological tests available for patients, and TNP animal models clearly do not reproduce the behavioral signs seen in the clinic, especially in the case of classical-TN. Hence, other than request imaging studies to detect possible lesions, tumors or vessel compressions along the trigeminal sensory system, the health professional depends almost strictly on the clinical criteria for the diagnosis.

Neuroimaging: Which neuroimaging techniques can be applied to investigate TNP?

The role of different parts of the brain in nociception has been revealed since the introduction of neuroimaging techniques in the early 1990s (4). Most of the methods currently applied do not measure the neuronal activity directly, but the changes in metabolism caused by the increase of neuronal activity in response to some stimulus (e.g., pain) (35). The most used neuroimaging techniques in the field of pain are: functional Magnetic Resonance Imaging (fMRI), magnetoencephalography (MEG), Positron Emission Tomography (PET) and Magnetic Resonance Spectroscopy (MRS). fMRI measures indirectly the neuronal activity with millimeter precision based on changes in the blood oxygenation level-dependent (BOLD) contrast, which relies on blood volume and blood flow. It allows a non-invasive investigation of function and dysfunction of the human brain (36). MEG measures directly current flows generated by neuronal synaptic activity with millisecond accuracy, but limited resolution. Although fMRI and MEG show neuronal activation in different ways, they are complementary and their integration is necessary to obtain the maximum information of brain activity during pain. PET applies radiolabeled active tracer along with mathematical models that allows the kinetic depiction of a bioactive tracer as it participates in a particular neuronal process in vivo. The measurement of the tracer concentration in the brain provides a three-dimensional image of the distribution of the biological process under study. This includes the capacity to quantify opioid receptor availability during challenges, such as pain, stress or even the introduction of a placebo, with corresponding physiological effects (37). MRS allows the detection of relatively small molecules, typically in concentrations of 0.5-nM. Its spectra provide information about metabolic pathways and it can be obtained by using several nuclei, including ^{1}H, ^{31}P, ^{19}F and others. However, ^{1}H is the most used for medical purposes because the high sensitivity of the ^{1}H nucleus, the large presence of this nucleus in most metabolites, and great availability of this isotope (38). H-MRS obtains chemical spectra from voxels within the human brain using radiofrequencies that excite protons (39). Based on the characteristic resonance frequency in the spectrum, particular molecules are identified. Once the spectra are acquired, they are analyzed to determine the relative concentrations of different molecules or metabolites of the central nervous system within the region of interest. The metabolites classically identified are: N-acetyl-aspartate (NAA), glutamate (Glu), creatine (Cr), choline (Cho), lactate, lipid, myoinositol, gamma-aminobutyric acid (GABA), and glutamine (Gln). Among them, Glu and GABA are of great interest, since they are components of excitatory and inhibitory neurotransmission, respectively.

Structural and functional neuroplasticity in TNP: How is the brain affected by trigeminal neuropathic pain?

The sensation of pain is frequently divided into a sensory-discriminative component and an affective-motivational component (40). The sensory-discriminative component of pain provides information about the location, modality, and intensity of painful stimuli. Its processing results in preferential activation of the lateral thalamus, somatosensory cortices (S1 and S2) and posterior insula (41). Conversely, the affective-motivational component of pain responds to the emotional responses provoked by pain, including feelings like suffering, fear, sadness, and anxiety. This emotional element of pain activates the anterior cingulate and insular cortices, which activate other components of the limbic system, such as the medial and dorsolateral prefrontal cortex that play a role in focusing attention to the stimuli (41, 42).

The cortical network involved in the processing of pain has been demonstrated by some previous studies. This network is frequently referred as pain neuromatrix (43, 44), a term derived from a former concept of neuromatrix (45, 46). The pain neuromatrix includes the primary (SI) and secondaru (SII) somatosensory cortices, motor cortex, cingulated cortex, frontal cortex and insula. Some recent studies have demonstrated structural and functional cortical changes associated to chronic pain, including fibromyalgia (47-50), chronic back pain (51), chronic tension type headache (52), migraine (53, 54) and trigeminal neuropathic pain (55, 56). However, there are still scarce clinical neuroimaging studies on trigeminal neuropathic pain disorders. In one of those studies, DaSilva, Becerra and colleagues (55) applied cortical surface reconstruction methods for MRI to compare the cortical thickness of patients with TNP affecting the right maxillary trigeminal division (V2) to healthy controls. They observed structural changes (cortical thickening or thinning) in the cortex of patients with TNP. Furthermore, the structural changes were colocalized with functional changes in most cortical regions associated with pain perception and behavior following brush-allodynic pain. Such dynamic functionally-driven changes in TNP included both cortical thickening and thinning in sensorimotor regions, and predominantly thinning in more anterior emotional regions, which correlated with the pain duration, age-at-onset, pain intensity and cortical activity. This cortical neuroplasticity in TNP patients may explain in part the chronification and treatment-resistance of their clinical pain. Another recent study applying fMRI in patients with classical trigeminal neuralgia showed activation of large parts of the pain neuromatrix even during non-painful stimulation of the affected area (in V2 or V3). This fact raises the possibility of hyperexcitability of the trigeminal system in patients with trigeminal neuropathic pain (56). One more relevant result from that study was the bilateral activation of S1, S2 and contralateral activation in the precentral cortex following stimulation of both sides in those patients who were submitted to retrogasserian radiofrequency thermocoagulation of the Gasserian ganglion (56) .

The thickness changes in the sensory cortex could be a result of chronic sensory stimulation provoked by chronic pain. This is in line with the results of a previous study that showed transient and selective thickening of the motion-visual areas (MT/V5) after learning to juggle (57). This suggests that overstimulation of neuronal systems in chronic pain may induce structural cortical changes that are colocalized with inefficient pain modulation by the opioidergic system at molecular level. In the following sections, we describe the most prominent functional and structural changes found in the brain of patients with trigeminal neuropathic pain. In addition, we provide a brief description of each cortical area significantly affected for this disorder.

Somatosensory Primary (SI) and Secondary (SII) cortices

The somatosensory cortex (Figure 1), which function is related to sensory-discriminative processing, is classically described as the anterior parietal cortex with its four subdivisions (putative Brodmann areas 3a, 3b, 1 and 2), all containing a somatotopic map of body regions. (58, 59).

The central sulcus and its bordering with the posterior wall of the the postcentral gyrus is usually considered the primary somatosensory cortex (SI) (putative 3b and 1). On the other hand, SII is localized lateroventrally to the postcentral gyrus, approximately between the anterior and posterior subcentral sulci on the operculum Rolandi (putative Brodmann area 43). It has been suggested that while SI might participate in the discriminative perception of pain intensity, SII would participate in the recognition of the noxious nature and also attention toward painful stimuli (60).

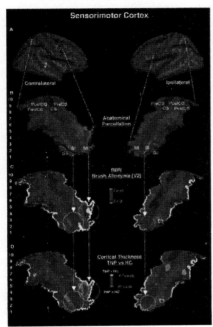

Figure 1. Sensorimotor cortex neuroplasticity in patients with TNP. Left side (a): *Panel A and B:* Regions of the sensorimotor cortex were segmented in ten equal vertical sections labeled from bottom to top, in an ascendant manner. *Panel C:* Average BOLD deactivations (dark-light blue) and activations (red-yellow) in the sensorimotor cortex during allodynic brush of the affected V2 of six TNP patients. *Panel D:* Differences in the cortical thickness between TNP patients and healthy controls along sections of the sensorimotor cortex. Right side: b. Structural and functional cortical changes in the sensorimotor cortex of patients with TNP. c. Summary of sensorimotor cortex functions (55).

There is a large representation of the face in the somatosensory cortex when compared with other body regions (61). The classical somatosensory homunculus originally drawn by Penfield described a right-side up orientation of the face (62). However, recent studies using fMRI have been revised this concept, and proposed an upside down orientation (63-65). As a result, the representation of the human trigeminal pain in the human somatosensory cortex exhibits an inverted representation of the face in a laminar sequence with V2 more rostral, V1 caudal and V3 medial (66).

Some recent studies have described functional and structural plasticity of the human somatosensory cortex in patients with chronic pain (54, 56, 67).

Comparing a group of patients with trigeminal neuropathic pain to a control group of healthy subjects DaSilva, Becerra and colleagues (55) observed bilateral thinning in the most caudal regions of the somatosensory cortex where the craniofacial structures are somatotopically represented (Figure 1). Furthermore, this bilateral thinning was colocalized with functional BOLD activations following brush allodynia of the affected area V2. Similar increased activity in the somatosensory cortex was also demonstrated in patients with classical trigeminal neuralgia after light tactile stimulation of the trigger zone (56) and after experimental tooth pain of upper and lower jaw in healthy subjects (68). It is interesting to notice that this pattern was inverted in the most rostral somatotopic regions of SI, including the hand/upper trunk somatotopic region that was significantly thicker bilaterally in TNP patients when compared to healthy controls (55). The thickening in the ipsilateral hand/upper trunk region was also spatially concurrent with BOLD deactivation during brush allodynia of V2. The thinning in the somatotopic facial regions of SI might be associated to overstimulation induced by neuropathic pain, while the thickening in the rostral neighboring regions of SI (somatotopic hand and trunk regions) are possibly related to either the increasing axial sprouting to the neighboring region, or activation of previously dormant cortico-cortical connections between those regions (69).

Motor cortex

According to the classical subdivision two distinct regions compose the motor cortex, the primary motor cortex (MI, putative Brodmann area 4), located anterior to the central sulcus and covering large parts of the precentral gyrus and the rostrally located non-primary motor cortex. Some anatomical observations support a further subdivision of the non-primary motor cortex in a premotor and a supplementary motor cortex. Similarly to the somatosensory cortex, the primary motor cortex encloses a somatotopic representation of several parts of the body (58).

Previous studies described motor cortex inhibition induced by pain. This process could be related to activation of C fibers and might be important to alert about possible nociceptive events that could occur near the painful region (70-72). DaSilva, Becerra and colleagues (55) did not find thickness changes in the orofacial area of MI when comparing patients with TNP and healthy controls. Nonetheless, they found significant thinning, colocalized with BOLD activation in the region that may represent the hand of MI contralateral to side the pain. Moreover, both structural and functional changes were also seen in pre-motor regions.

Recent studies have been demonstrating the benefits of motor cortex stimulation in some conditions of chronic pain, including pain of central origin (73), fibromyalgia (74, 75) and trigeminal pain. One possible explanation for the pain relief after motor cortex stimulation is that increased motor cortex activity could modulate abnormal thalamic activity via cortico-thalamic fibers. The secondary modulation of the thalamic nuclei might underlie the pain-relief function of motor cortex stimulation (42).

Latero-frontal cortex

The frontal cortex (Figure 2) is the part of the brain localized anterior to the central sulcus and superior to the lateral fissure.

Its complex morphology has been extensively studied. Based on the results of recent cytoarchitectonic studies, the region anterior to the precentral motor area can be divided as follows: ventrolateral prefrontal cortex (putative Brodmann areas 44,45 and 47/12); orbital frontal cortex (putative Brodmann areas 11, 13 and 14); frontopolar cortex (putative Brodmann area 10); dorsolateral prefrontal cortex (putative areas 8; 9; 9/46 and 46) and medial frontal cortex (putative Brodmann areas 24; 25 and 32) (58). Neuroimaging studies reported that the activity of the frontal cortex is related to the processing of reward and punishment. This activity is observed in some situations like: decision making, addiction, and pain (76-78). Specifically, the orbitofrontal cortex can be anatomically divided into a medial segment, which activity is associated to monitoring the reward value of many different reinforcers; and the lateral part, which activity is linked to the evaluation of the punishment value of reinforcers (e.g., pain) (78).

Patients with TNP group exhibited thinning in the frontal middle gyri (figure 2) extending to the correspondent sulci bilaterally (putative BA10), in the anterior frontal gyrus in the contralateral side to the pain and in the ipsilateral posterior orbital gyrus (putative BA 47/12). All the areas of cortical thinning in the frontal cortex were precisely colocalized with BOLD deactivation following brush allodynic stimulation (55). The cortical thinning found in the frontal cortex might be associated with the underlying change in affective-emotional processing that can participate of comorbid changes seen in chronic pain patients (55).

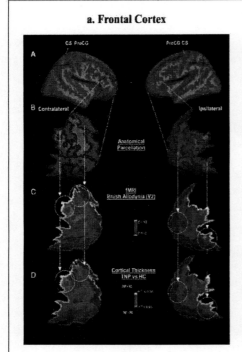

Figure 2. Frontal cortex neuroplasticity in patients with TNP. Left side (a): *Panel A and B:* The latero-frontal cortex was parcellated in seven regions. *Panel C:* Average BOLD deactivations (dark-light blue) and activations (red-yellow) in the frontal cortex during allodynic brush of the affected V2 of six TNP patients. *Panel D:* Differences in the cortical thickness between TNP patients and healthy controls along sections of the frontal cortex. Right side: b. Structural and functional cortical changes in the frontal cortex of patients with TNP. c. Summary of the main functions related to the frontal cortex (55).

In another recent study involving patients with classical trigeminal neuralgia, bilateral activation of the prefrontal cortex was observed after tactile stimulation of the trigger zone (56). Conversely, patients with acute, left-sided, post-molar extraction (surgical) pain showed significantly reduced responses to experimental heat pain (applied to the right hand) in the anterior cingulate, pre-frontal medial and orbito-frontal cortices when measured by positron emission tomography (79).

Dorsolateral Prefrontal Cortex (DLPFC)

The dorsolateral prefrontal cortex is related to executive functions, memory and attention. It comprises the superior and middle frontal gyri, and extends medially to the paracingulate sulcus (putative Brodmann areas 8, 9 and 46) (58). The area 9 occupies part of the superior frontal gyrus and part of the middle frontal gyrus. However, recent studies of comparative anatomy described different cytoarchitectures between these two territories of the area 9. Therefore, the original area 9 can be divided in two other regions: the part that belongs to the superior frontal gyrus (area 9) and the part that lies on the middle frontal gyrus, named area 9/46 according to this subdivision (80, 81)

Neuroimaging studies suggest an important role of the DLPFC in the mechanisms of mood disorders and chronic pain (82-84). DaSilva, Becerra and colleagues (55) demonstrated bilateral thinning mainly in the frontal inferior sulci (putative BA 9/46 ventral) of DLPFC in patients with TNP. This structural adaptation was also colocalized with sparse BOLD activations and deactivations. Similar cortical changes in the DLPFC were found in a study involving patients with chronic back pain (85). In addition, another study showed decrease gray-matter volume in the DLPFC of chronic pain patients associated to decreased levels of N-acetylaspartate, a common marker of neurodegenerative disorders (86). One possible explanation for the cortical thickness changes in the DLPFC could be chronic stress causing overuse and atrophy in the DLPFC. The inputs for this modulation could probably come from the medial thalamic nucleus, as well as from primary sensory regions. Dysfunction of DLPFC might play a role in the difficulties that chronic pain patients have, and also intensify their co-morbid clinical problems (e.g. depression and anxiety) (55).

Cingulate cortex

The cingulate gyrus (Figure 3) is the most pronounced cortical structure on the medial aspect of the human brain.

It extends from the lamina terminalis rostral to the anterior comissure, surrounding the corpus callosum (58, 87) According to general view, the cingulate cortex is a crucial region for emotion (88). The neurobiological model integrating cytoarchitecture, afferent connections, regional composition and functional properties divide the cingulate cortex in four distinct regions: Anterior Cingulate Cortex (ACC) related to emotion (includes Brodmann areas 25, 33, 24 and 32); Midcingulate Cortex (MCC) associated with response selection and subdivided in anterior and posterior (Brodmann areas 33', 24', 24d and 32'); Posterior Cingulate Cortex (PCC) involved in personal orientation and subdivided in dorsal and ventral (Brodmann areas 23 and 31) and Retrosplenial Cortex (RSC) responsible for memory formation/access (Brodmann areas 29 and 30).

In the study of DaSilva, Becerra and colleagues (55) the posterior subdivision of midcingulate cortex (pMCC) contralateral to the side of pain (postulated BA 24/31) showed significant thinning in TNP patients when compared to the same region in healthy subjects (Figure 3).

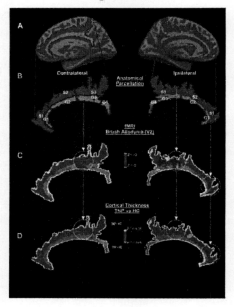

Figure 3. Cingulate cortex neuroplasticity in patients with TNP. Left side (a): *Panel A and B:* The cingulate cortex was segmented in seven regions. *Panel C:* Average BOLD deactivations (dark-light blue) and activations (red-yellow) in the cingulate cortex during allodynic brush of the affected V2 of six TNP patients. *Panel D:* Differences in the cortical thickness between TNP patients and healthy controls along sections of the cingulate cortex. Right side: b. Structural and functional cortical changes in the cingulate cortex of patients with TNP. c. Summary of the main functions related to the cingulate cortex (55).

This thinning spatially coincided with BOLD deactivation during allodynic brush stimulation of the affected V2 region. This area is part of the motor cingulate cortex, adjacent to the supplementary motor cortex (SMA) and has a large interaction with the posterior parietal cortex. The function of the pMCC in pain is more related to the skeletomotor orientation in reaction to the neuropathic pain than to the nociceptive processing (55). In addition, the involvement of this area in trigeminal pain was described in other studies (79, 83). Different from the pMCC, the antero-mid cingulate sulcus (putative BA 32'/24') showed cortical thickening ipsilateral to allodynic pain in TNP patients, when compared to healthy controls (55). This region has connections to the amygdala and may be involved in fear avoidance of the perception of TNP. The retrosplenial cortex a region that is implicated with topographic and topokinetic memory (58) showed a thinning contralateral to the side of the pain. However, these structural findings did not spatially coincided with the BOLD changes. Finally, there was a cortical thinning that was adjacent to BOLD activation in the anterior cingulate cortex gyrus (putative BA 33/24) ipsilateral to the pain, a region considered to play an important role in affective-motivational processing (88).

Insula

The insular cortex or insula (Figure 4) is located in the centre of the cerebral hemisphere, covered by the frontal and lateral opercula as well as temporal lobe and consequently hidden from the view in the lateral fissure (58, 87).

It has been divided in two regions: anterior and posterior insula (89). A large number of structures are connected to the insula, including: primary and secondary somatosensory areas (SI and SII), Anterior Cingulate Cortex (ACC), amygdaloid body, prefrontal cortex, superior temporal gyrus, orbitofrontal cortex, frontal operculum, parietal operculum, primary auditory cortex, auditory association cortex, visual association cortex, olfactory bulb, hippocampus, entorhinal cortex and motor cortex (87, 90). The functions associated to the insular cortex are: processing of visceral sensory, vestibular function, attention, pain, emotion, verbal, motor and musical information as well as gustatory, olfactory, visual, auditory and tactile processing (87).

The role of the insular cortex in the processing of pain input is supported by several studies. In fact, the insula receives information from a direct thalamo-insular connection and might be a site of sensory and affective integration (89).

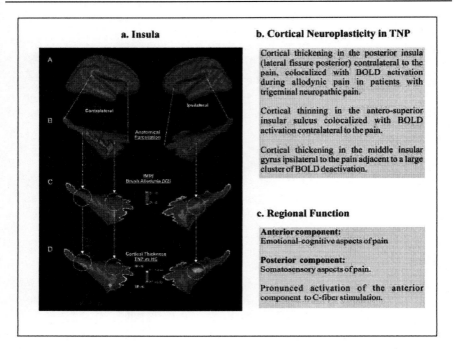

Figure 4. Insula cortex neuroplasticity in patients with TNP. Left side (a): *Panel A and B:* The insula was subdivided in seven parcellated regions along the lateral fissure posterior, insular superior and inferior sulci and the insular gyrus. *Panel C:* Average BOLD deactivations (dark-light blue) and activations (red-yellow) in the insula during allodynic brush of the affected V2 of six TNP patients. *Panel D:* Differences in the cortical thickness between TNP patients and healthy controls along sections of the insula. Right side: b. Structural and functional cortical changes in the insular cortex of patients with TNP. c. Summary of the insula functions (55).

Moreover, its somatotopic organization was recently demonstrated with respect to muscle and cutaneous pain, and that this organization is further separated according to the tissue in which the pain originates (91, 92). Cortical thickening was seen in the posterior insula (lateral fissure posterior) contralateral to the neuropathic pain in TNP patients when compared to a heath control group. This thickening was colocalized with BOLD activation following allodynic stimulation of the affected area. In the same side, a cortical thinning was found in the antero-superior insula when compared to the same area in the control group, which was only adjacent to BOLD activation (figure 4). Elevated BOLD signals were also found in the anterior insula after light tactile stimulation of the trigger zone in patients with classical trigeminal neuralgia (41) and after experimental tooth pain in the upper and lower jaw

(68) It seems that the anterior insula process more detailed aspects of pain, including the distinction between clinical and experimental nature of pain (93), visceromotor and autonomic responses (94) and more affective-motivational qualities of pain, including expectation (43) and unpleasantness (95). The cortical thinning in the anterior insula may represent a tendency of chronic pain to induce thinning in regions related to affective-motivational process (55). Cortical thickening was also noticed in the middle insular gyrus ipsilateral side to the pain in TNP when compared to health subjects, which was adjacent to a large cluster of BOLD deactivation that extended to more anterior regions.

Trigeminal Sensory input: How does afferent fibers' input influence cortical reorganization in neuropathic pain disorders?

Experimental pain commonly activates the primary and secondary somatosensory cortex (SI and SII), insula and anterior cingulate cortex (96, 97). This activation depends on the stimulus type, size, intensity and location, as well as other factors that contribute to the discriminative, affective and cognitive aspects of pain (98, 99). For instance, administration of capsaicin to the forehead, evoking a long-lasting pain mediated mainly by C fibers, activates the anterior insula and cingulate cortices bilaterally (100). These anterior areas are usually correlated with affective processing of pain. Another study used fMRI to investigate brain activation after selective activation of $A\delta$ and C fibers in tiny areas of the skin. The results revealed that the right anterior insula together with parts of the frontal operculum and left insula are significantly more activated in response to C-fiber stimulation than $A\delta$-fiber stimulation and suggest that C fibers are more important for interoceptive and homeostatic functions than $A\delta$ fibers (101). Conversely, when painful stimulus primarily conducted by $A\delta$ fibers is applied to the hand, strong activation is also observed in the contra-lateral SI, and often bilateral SII, cingulate, insular and prefrontal cortices (102). There is a debate over the role of SI and SII, in addition to the other cortical structures, regarding the processing of each painful stimulus aspect, mainly due to the limited temporal resolution of the techniques utilized (fMRI and PET) (59). MEG has been recently employed in experimental studies of pain (35, 103). MEG data not only show temporal differences between the first pain and second pain, but also cortical sequential phase-locked activations correlated with each other (104). When a painful laser stimulus is applied to the dorsum of the hand, both pain sensations, first

($A\delta$) and second pain (C fiber), have unique features under MEG analysis (105). Although SII is equally activated, the first pain sensation is strongly correlated with SI activation, and the second pain with that of the anterior cingulate cortex. Nevertheless, it seems that SI and SII code pain intensity in a different way. The activation in SI is directly proportionate to stimulus intensity, and activation in SII has an "all-or-none-like" characteristic, responding to pain intensity only after a certain threshold (60)

Using PET Hsieh and colleagues (106) showed that in mononeuropathy patients there is positive activation of affective-motivational cortical areas including cingulate, and prefrontal cortex, but no changes in the somatosensory cortex. However, when time-resolution of the neuroimaging tool increases, more of the earlier cortical mechanisms of neuropathic pain are discriminated. Maihofner and colleagues (107) studied a patient with femoral neuropathic pain with allodynic skin area that when lightly brushed evoked a shooting pain followed by burning sensation. MEG imaging of the patient showed strong and laterally displaced activation in the SI compared to the unaffected side stimulation. A peak activation located in the posterior cingulate cortex was detected with a fast velocity range suggestive of $A\beta$ fiber involvement. This persistent dysfunctional influence of $A\beta$ and C fibers in cortical activity that takes place in neuropathic pain patients seems to induce not only functional, but structural neuroplasticity in their brains.

Conclusion and perspectives

Recent neuroimaging data demonstrate that the chronic suffering from TNP leads to gray matter reorganization that occurs at multiple intrinsic subcortical and cortical systems associated with sensory and emotional changes. This maladaptive remodeling activity may be responsible for the persistence of the illness and pain modulatory dysfunction in those patients. One potential insight gained from those studies may relate to the difficulty in treating neuropathic pain that simple treatment and removal of the peripheral and initial cause do not account for functional and structural changes in multiple cortical regions associated with pain perception and modulation. And even tough new pharmacologic treatments are emerging; they have been unable to target specifically those dysfunctional brain regions. Novel non-invasive stimulation methods are promising therapies that can safely and directly modulate the cortical regions affected by TNP with significant pain relief, but more studies are needed to investigate their lasting neuroplastic outcome.

Acknowledgment

This work was supported by the following grants: Dr. DaSilva was supported by NIH K23 NS062946, DANA Foundation's Brain and Immuno-imaging award, and MICHR Clinical Trial Planning Program/CTSA high-tech funding UL1RR024986, University of Michigan. Dr. Santos was supported by the Coordenação de Aperfeiçoamento de Pessoal de Nível Superior (CAPES), Brazil and by the University of Michigan, Ann Arbor, US.

References

[1]   Taxonomy ITFo. Classification of Chronic Pain. 2nd ed. Seattle: IASP Press, 1994.

[2]   Apkarian AV, Baliki MN, Geha PY. Towards a theory of chronic pain. Prog Neurobiol 2009;87:81-97.

[3]   Dieleman J, Kerklaan J, Huygen F, Bouma P, Sturkenboom M. Incidence rates and treatment of neuropathic pain conditions in the general population. Pain 2008;137:681-8.

[4]   Wall PD, McMahon SB, Koltzenburg M. Wall and Melzack's textbook of pain. Philadelphia: Elsevier/Churchill Livingstone, 2006.

[5]   Bennett G. Neuropathic pain in the orofacial region: clinical and research challenges. J Orofac Pain 2004;18:281-6.

[6]   Okeson JP, Bell WE. Bell's orofacial pains: the clinical management of orofacial pain. Chicago: Quintessence, 2005.

[7]   Katusic S, Beard C, Bergstralh E, Kurland L. Incidence and clinical features of trigeminal neuralgia, Rochester, Minnesota, 1945-1984. Ann Neurol 1990;27:89-95.

[8]   Bennetto L, Patel N, Fuller G. Trigeminal neuralgia and its management. BMJ 2007;334:201-5.

[9]   Hall G, Carroll D, Parry D, McQuay H. Epidemiology and treatment of neuropathic pain: the UK primary care perspective. Pain 2006;122:156-62.

[10]   Hall G, Carroll D, McQuay H. Primary care incidence and treatment of four neuropathic pain conditions: a descriptive study, 2002-2005. BMC Fam Pract 2008;9:1-9.

[11]   Koopman J, Dieleman J, Huygen F, de Mos M, Martin C, Sturkenboom M. Incidence of facial pain in the general population. Pain 2009;147:122-7.

[12]   Zakrzewska JM. Facial pain: neurological and non-neurological. J Neurol Neurosurg Psychiatry 2002;72 Suppl 2:ii27-32.

[13]   Sindou M, Howeidy T, Acevedo G. Anatomical observations during microvascular decompression for idiopathic trigeminal neuralgia (with correlations between topography of pain and site of the neurovascular conflict). Prospective study in a series of 579 patients. Acta Neurochirurgica 2002;144:1-13.

[14]   de Leeuw R, editor. Orofacial pain: guidelines for assessment, diagnosis, and management. Chicago: Quintessence, 2008.

[15]   Zakrzewska J. Trigeminal Neuralgia. London: W. B. Saunders, 1995.
[16]   Türp J, Gobetti J. Trigeminal neuralgia versus atypical facial pain. A review of the literature and case report. Oral Surg Oral Med Oral Pathol Oral Radiol Endod 1996;81:424-32.
[17]   Cusick J. Atypical trigeminal neuralgia. JAMA 1981;245:2328-9.
[18]   Tancioni F, Gaetani P, Villani L, Zappoli F, Rodriguez Y, Baena R. Neurinoma of the trigeminal root and atypical trigeminal neuralgia: case report and review of the literature. Surg Neurol 1995;44:36-42.
[19]   Silberstein S, Olesen J, Bousser M, Diener H, Dodick D, First M, et al. The International Classification of Headache Disorders, 2nd Edition (ICHD-II)--revision of criteria for 8.2 Medication-overuse headache. Cephalalgia 2005;25:460-5.
[20]   Watson C, Oaklander A. Postherpetic neuralgia. Pain Pract 2002;2:295-307.
[21]   Weinberg J. Herpes zoster: epidemiology, natural history, and common complications. J Am Acad Dermatol 2007;57(6 Suppl):S130-5.
[22]   Katz J, Cooper E, Walther R, Sweeney E, Dworkin R. Acute pain in herpes zoster and its impact on health-related quality of life. Clin Infect Dis 2004;39:342-8.
[23]   Insinga R, Itzler R, Pellissier J, Saddier P, Nikas A. The incidence of herpes zoster in a United States administrative database. J Gen Intern Med 2005;20:748-53.
[24]   Hope-Simpson R. The nature of herpes zoster: a long-term study and a new hypothesis. Proc R Soc Med 1965;58:9-20.
[25]   de Leeuw R, editor. Orofacial pain: guidelines for assessment, diagnosis, and management. Chicago: Quintessence, 2008.
[26]   Arvin AM, Gershon AA, Foundation VZVR. Varicella-zoster virus: virology and clinical management. Cambridge: Cambridge University Press, 2000.
[27]   Delaney A, Colvin LA, Fallon MT, Dalziel RG, Mitchell R, Fleetwood-Walker SM. Postherpetic neuralgia: from preclinical models to the clinic. Neurotherapeutics 2009;6:630-7.
[28]   Dworkin RH, Gnann JW, Jr., Oaklander AL, Raja SN, Schmader KE, Whitley RJ. Diagnosis and assessment of pain associated with herpes zoster and postherpetic neuralgia. J Pain 2008;9(1 Suppl 1):S37-44.
[29]   Burgoon CJ, Burgoon J, Baldridge G. The natural history of herpes zoster. J Am Med Assoc 1957;164:265-9.
[30]   De Moragas J, Kierland R. The outcome of patients with herpes zoster. AMA Arch Derm 1957;75:193-6.
[31]   Cooper M. The epidemiology of herpes zoster. Eye 1987;1(Pt3):413-21.
[32]   Brown G. Herpes zoster: correlation of age, sex, distribution, neuralgia, and associated disorders. South Med J 1976;69:576-8.
[33]   Watson P, Evans R. Postherpetic neuralgia. A review. Arch Neurol 1986;43:836-40.
[34]   Oaklander A. The density of remaining nerve endings in human skin with and without postherpetic neuralgia after shingles. Pain 2001;92:139-45.
[35]   Bromm B. Brain images of pain. News Physiol Sci 2001;16:244-9.
[36]   Heeger D, Ress D. What does fMRI tell us about neuronal activity? Nat Rev Neurosci 2002;3:142-51.

[37] Zubieta J, Bueller J, Jackson L, Scott D, Xu Y, Koeppe R, et al. Placebo effects mediated by endogenous opioid activity on mu-opioid receptors. J Neurosci 2005;25:7754-62.

[38] Van Der Graaf M. In vivo magnetic resonance spectroscopy: basic methodology and clinical applications. Eur Biophys J 2010;39:527-40.

[39] Ross A, Sachdev P. Magnetic resonance spectroscopy in cognitive research. Brain Res Brain Res Rev 2004;44:83-102.

[40] Treede R, Kenshalo D, Gracely R, Jones A. The cortical representation of pain. Pain 1999;79:105-11.

[41] Moisset X, Bouhassira D. Functional brain imaging of trigeminal neuralgia. Eur J Pain 2010 july.

[42] Zaghi S, Heine N, Fregni F. Brain stimulation for the treatment of pain: A review of costs, clinical effects, and mechanisms of treatment for three different central neuromodulatory approaches. J Pain Manag 2009;2:339-52.

[43] Ploghaus A, Tracey I, Gati J, Clare S, Menon R, Matthews P, et al. Dissociating pain from its anticipation in the human brain. Science 1999;284:1979-81.

[44] Iannetti G, Mouraux A. From the neuromatrix to the pain matrix (and back). Exp Brain Res 2010;205:1-12.

[45] Melzack R. Evolution of the neuromatrix theory of pain. The Prithvi Raj Lecture: presented at the third World Congress of World Institute of Pain, Barcelona 2004. Pain Pract 2005;5:85-94.

[46] Melzack R. Labat lecture. Phantom limbs. Reg Anesth 1989;14:208-11.

[47] Kuchinad A, Schweinhardt P, Seminowicz D, Wood P, Chizh B, Bushnell M. Accelerated brain gray matter loss in fibromyalgia patients: premature aging of the brain? J Neurosci 2007;27:4004-7.

[48] Hsu M, Harris R, Sundgren P, Welsh R, Fernandes C, Clauw D, et al. No consistent difference in gray matter volume between individuals with fibromyalgia and age-matched healthy subjects when controlling for affective disorder. Pain 2009;143:262-7.

[49] Schmidt-Wilcke T, Luerding R, Weigand T, Jürgens T, Schuierer G, Leinisch E, et al. Striatal grey matter increase in patients suffering from fibromyalgia--a voxel-based morphometry study. Pain 2007;(132 Suppl 1):S109-16.

[50] Lutz J, Jäger L, de Quervain D, Krauseneck T, Padberg F, Wichnalek M, et al. White and gray matter abnormalities in the brain of patients with fibromyalgia: a diffusion-tensor and volumetric imaging study. Arthritis Rheum 2008;58:3960-9.

[51] Schmidt-Wilcke T, Leinisch E, Gänssbauer S, Draganski B, Bogdahn U, Altmeppen J, et al. Affective components and intensity of pain correlate with structural differences in gray matter in chronic back pain patients. Pain 2006;125:89-97.

[52] Schmidt-Wilcke T, Leinisch E, Straube A, Kämpfe N, Draganski B, Diener H, et al. Gray matter decrease in patients with chronic tension type headache. Neurology 2005;65:1483-6.

[53] Kim J, Suh S, Seol H, Oh K, Seo W, Yu S, et al. Regional grey matter changes in patients with migraine: a voxel-based morphometry study. Cephalalgia 2008;28:598-604.

[54] DaSilva A, Granziera C, Snyder J, Hadjikhani N. Thickening in the somatosensory cortex of patients with migraine. Neurology 2007;69:1990-5.

[55] DaSilva AF, Becerra L, Pendse G, Chizh B, Tully S, Borsook D. Colocalized structural and functional changes in the cortex of patients with trigeminal neuropathic pain. PLoS One 2008;3:e3396.

[56] Moisset X, Villain N, Ducreux D, Serrie A, Cunin G, Valade D, et al. Functional brain imaging of trigeminal neuralgia. Eur J Pain 2010 July.

[57] Draganski B, Gaser C, Busch V, Schuierer G, Bogdahn U, May A. Neuroplasticity: changes in grey matter induced by training. Nature 2004;427:311-2.

[58] Paxinos G, Mai JrK. The Human nervous system. San Diego: Elsevier Academic Press, 2004.

[59] Bushnell M, Duncan G, Hofbauer R, Ha B, Chen J, Carrier B. Pain perception: is there a role for primary somatosensory cortex? Proc Natl Acad Sci U S A 1999;96:7705-9.

[60] Timmermann L, Ploner M, Haucke K, Schmitz F, Baltissen R, Schnitzler A. Differential coding of pain intensity in the human primary and secondary somatosensory cortex. J Neurophysiol 2001;86:1499-503.

[61] Borsook D, DaSilva A, Ploghaus A, Becerra L. Specific and somatotopic functional magnetic resonance imaging activation in the trigeminal ganglion by brush and noxious heat. J Neurosci 2003;23:7897-903.

[62] Wilder P, Edwin B. Somatotopic motor and sensory representation in the cerebral cortex of man as studied by electrical stimulation. Brain 1937;60:389-433.

[63] Pons T, Garraghty P, Ommaya A, Kaas J, Taub E, Mishkin M. Massive cortical reorganization after sensory deafferentation in adult macaques. Science 1991;252:1857-60.

[64] Servos P, Engel S, Gati J, Menon R. fMRI evidence for an inverted face representation in human somatosensory cortex. Neuroreport 1999;10:1393-5.

[65] Yang T, Gallen C, Schwartz B, Bloom F. Noninvasive somatosensory homunculus mapping in humans by using a large-array biomagnetometer. Proc Natl Acad Sci U S A 1993;90:3098-102.

[66] DaSilva A, Becerra L, Makris N, Strassman A, Gonzalez R, Geatrakis N, et al. Somatotopic activation in the human trigeminal pain pathway. J Neurosci 2002;22:8183-92.

[67] Granziera C, DaSilva A, Snyder J, Tuch D, Hadjikhani N. Anatomical alterations of the visual motion processing network in migraine with and without aura. PLoS Med 2006;3:e402.

[68] Weigelt A, Terekhin P, Kemppainen P, Dörfler A, Forster C. The representation of experimental tooth pain from upper and lower jaws in the human trigeminal pathway. Pain 2010;149:529-38.

[69] Clarey J, Tweedale R, Calford M. Interhemispheric modulation of somatosensory receptive fields: evidence for plasticity in primary somatosensory cortex. Cereb Cortex 1996;6:196-206.

[70] Romaniello A, Cruccu G, McMillan AS, Arendt-Nielsen L, Svensson P. Effect of experimental pain from trigeminal muscle and skin on motor cortex excitability in humans. Brain Res 2000;882:120-7.

Functional and structural cortical neuroplasticity ...

[71] Farina S, Valeriani M, Rosso T, Aglioti S, Tamburin S, Fiaschi A, et al. Transient inhibition of the human motor cortex by capsaicin-induced pain. A study with transcranial magnetic stimulation. Neurosci Lett 2001;314:97-101.

[72] Svensson P, Miles TS, McKay D, Ridding MC. Suppression of motor evoked potentials in a hand muscle following prolonged painful stimulation. Eur J Pain 2003;7:55-62.

[73] Fregni F, Boggio P, Lima M, Ferreira M, Wagner T, Rigonatti S, et al. A sham-controlled, phase II trial of transcranial direct current stimulation for the treatment of central pain in traumatic spinal cord injury. Pain 2006;122:197-209.

[74] Fregni F, Gimenes R, Valle AC, Ferreira MJ, Rocha RR, Natalle L, et al. A randomized, sham-controlled, proof of principle study of transcranial direct current stimulation for the treatment of pain in fibromyalgia. Arthritis Rheum 2006;54:3988-98.

[75] Roizenblatt S, Fregni F, Gimenez R, Wetzel T, Rigonatti SP, Tufik S, et al. Site-specific effects of transcranial direct current stimulation on sleep and pain in fibromyalgia: a randomized, sham-controlled study. Pain Pract 2007;7:297-306.

[76] Carlsson K, Andersson J, Petrovic P, Petersson K, Ohman A, Ingvar M. Predictability modulates the affective and sensory-discriminative neural processing of pain. Neuroimage 2006;32:1804-14.

[77] Goldstein R, Tomasi D, Rajaram S, Cottone L, Zhang L, Maloney T, et al. Role of the anterior cingulate and medial orbitofrontal cortex in processing drug cues in cocaine addiction. Neuroscience 2007;144:1153-9.

[78] Tobler P, O'Doherty J, Dolan R, Schultz W. Reward value coding distinct from risk attitude-related uncertainty coding in human reward systems. J Neurophysiol 2007;97:1621-32.

[79] Derbyshire S, Jones A, Collins M, Feinmann C, Harris M. Cerebral responses to pain in patients suffering acute post-dental extraction pain measured by positron emission tomography (PET). Eur J Pain 1999;3:103-13.

[80] Petrides M, Pandya DN. Dorsolateral prefrontal cortex: comparative cytoarchitectonic analysis in the human and the macaque brain and corticocortical connection patterns. Eur J Neurosci 1999;11:1011-36.

[81] Petrides M, Pandya DN. Comparative cytoarchitectonic analysis of the human and the macaque ventrolateral prefrontal cortex and corticocortical connection patterns in the monkey. Eur J Neurosci 2002;16:291-310.

[82] Peyron R, García-Larrea L, Grégoire M, Convers P, Lavenne F, Veyre L, et al. Allodynia after lateral-medullary (Wallenberg) infarct. A PET study. Brain 1998;121(Pt2):345-56.

[83] Hsieh J, Hannerz J, Ingvar M. Right-lateralised central processing for pain of nitroglycerin-induced cluster headache. Pain 1996;67:59-68.

[84] Grachev I, Ramachandran T, Thomas P, Szeverenyi N, Fredrickson B. Association between dorsolateral prefrontal N-acetyl aspartate and depression in chronic back pain: an in vivo proton magnetic resonance spectroscopy study. J Neural Transm 2003;110:287-312.

128 Marcos FH DosSantos and Alexandre F DaSilva

[85] Apkarian A, Sosa Y, Sonty S, Levy R, Harden R, Parrish T, et al. Chronic back pain is associated with decreased prefrontal and thalamic gray matter density. J Neurosci 2004;24:10410-5.
[86] Grachev I, Fredrickson B, Apkarian A. Brain chemistry reflects dual states of pain and anxiety in chronic low back pain. J Neural Transm 2002;109:1309-34.
[87] Nagai M, Kishi K, Kato S. Insular cortex and neuropsychiatric disorders: a review of recent literature. Eur Psychiatry 2007;22:387-94.
[88] Vogt B. Pain and emotion interactions in subregions of the cingulate gyrus. Nat Rev Neurosci 2005;6:533-44.
[89] Brooks J, Tracey I. The insula: a multidimensional integration site for pain. Pain 2007;128:1-2.
[90] Augustine J. Circuitry and functional aspects of the insular lobe in primates including humans. Brain Res Brain Res Rev 1996;22:229-44.
[91] Ostrowsky K, Magnin M, Ryvlin P, Isnard J, Guenot M, Mauguière F. Representation of pain and somatic sensation in the human insula: a study of responses to direct electrical cortical stimulation. Cereb Cortex 2002;12:376-85.
[92] Henderson L, Gandevia S, Macefield V. Somatotopic organization of the processing of muscle and cutaneous pain in the left and right insula cortex: a single-trial fMRI study. Pain 2007;128:20-30.
[93] Schweinhardt P, Glynn C, Brooks J, McQuay H, Jack T, Chessell I, et al. An fMRI study of cerebral processing of brush-evoked allodynia in neuropathic pain patients. Neuroimage 2006;32:256-65.
[94] Ostrowsky K, Isnard J, Ryvlin P, Guénot M, Fischer C, Mauguière F. Functional mapping of the insular cortex: clinical implication in temporal lobe epilepsy. Epilepsia 2000;41:681-6.
[95] Schreckenberger M, Siessmeier T, Viertmann A, Landvogt C, Buchholz H, Rolke R, et al. The unpleasantness of tonic pain is encoded by the insular cortex. Neurology 2005;64:1175-83.
[96] Casey KL. Concepts of pain mechanisms: the contribution of functional imaging of the human brain. Prog Brain Res 2000;129:277-87.
[97] Casey KL BM. Pain Imaging. Progress in Pain Research and Management. Seattle: IASP Press, 2000.
[98] Apkarian AV, Gelnar PA, Krauss BR, Szeverenyi NM. Cortical responses to thermal pain depend on stimulus size: a functional MRI study. J Neurophysiol 2000;83:3113-22.
[99] Villemure C, Bushnell MC. Cognitive modulation of pain: how do attention and emotion influence pain processing? Pain 2002;95:195-9.
[100] May A, Kaube H, Buchel C, Eichten C, Rijntjes M, Juptner M, et al. Experimental cranial pain elicited by capsaicin: a PET study. Pain 1998;74:61-6.
[101] Weiss T, Straube T, Boettcher J, Hecht H, Spohn D, Miltner W. Brain activation upon selective stimulation of cutaneous C- and Adelta-fibers. Neuroimage 2008;41:1372-81.
[102] Creac'h C, Henry P, Caille JM, Allard M. Functional MR imaging analysis of pain-related brain activation after acute mechanical stimulation. AJNR Am J Neuroradiol 2000;21:1402-6.

Functional and structural cortical neuroplasticity ... 129

[103] Arendt-Nielsen L, Yamasaki H, Nielsen J, Naka D, Kakigi R. Magnetoencephalographic responses to painful impact stimulation. Brain Res 1999;839:203-8.

[104] Simoes C, Jensen O, Parkkonen L, Hari R. Phase locking between human primary and secondary somatosensory cortices. Proc Natl Acad Sci U S A 2003;100:2691-4.

[105] Ploner M, Gross J, Timmermann L, Schnitzler A. Cortical representation of first and second pain sensation in humans. Proc Natl Acad Sci U S A 2002;99:12444-8.

[106] Hsieh JC, Belfrage M, Stone-Elander S, Hansson P, Ingvar M. Central representation of chronic ongoing neuropathic pain studied by positron emission tomography. Pain 1995;63:225-36.

[107] Maihofner C, Neundorfer B, Stefan H, Handwerker HO. Cortical processing of brush-evoked allodynia. Neuroreport 2003;14:785-9.

Chapter VIII

Brain Stimulation for the treatment of neuropathic facial pain

Helena Knotkova, PhD[*,1,2]*, Arash Nafissi, MD*[1,3]*,*
Eliah Soto, MD[1]*, Dirk Rasche, MD*[4]
and Ricardo A Cruciani, MD, PhD[1,2,5]

[1]Institute for Non-invasive Brain Stimulation, Research Division,
Department of Pain Medicine and Palliative Care,
Beth Israel Medical Center, New York, New York, US
[2]Department of Neurology, Albert Einstein College of Medicine,
Bronx, New York, US
[3]Department of Rehabilitation Medicine, New York University Medical
Center, New York, New York, US
[4]Department of Neurosurgery, University of Lübeck, Lübeck, Germany;
[5]Department of Anesthesiology, Albert Einstein College of Medicine,
Bronx, New York, US

[*] Correspondence: Helena Knotkova, PhD, INBSNY, Department of Pain Medicine and Palliative Care, 120 E 16th Str., 12th fl., Beth Israel Medical Center, New York, NY, 10003, United States of America. E-mail: HKnotkov@chpnet.org

Abstract

In the past two decades, cutting edge technologies such as transcranial magnetic stimulation (TMS), transcranial direct current stimulation (tDCS), epidural motor cortex stimulation (MCS) and deep brain stimulation (DBS), have been shown to be effective tools for modulation of neural excitability. Since then, these techniques have been explored for the management of numerous medical conditions, including pain management. The rationale for the use of brain stimulation in the treatment of pain is based on recent findings that patients with various chronic pain syndromes present with pathological changes in brain excitability, and that modulation of such changes can be paralleled by pain relief. TMS, tDCS, MCS or DBS have been shown to be effective tools for modulation of neural excitability, and have been in the past two decades implemented into research and clinical practice of pain management in patients with various difficult-to-treat neuropathic pain syndromes. Findings from controlled trials indicate that brain stimulation techniques have significant clinical potential in the treatment of chronic pain in selected patient-populations. This chapter reviews and discusses the use of invasive- and non-invasive brain stimulation in the treatment of neuropathic facial pain.

Presented information can serve as a useful resource for future brain-stimulation studies and for implementation of novel non-pharmacological techniques into management of chronic facial pain.

Introduction

In the past two decades, brain stimulation techniques have been shown to be effective tools for modulation of neural excitability and have been explored in numerous medical fields and applications, including pain management. The introduction of invasive- as well as non-invasive- brain stimulation methods into the research and treatment of chronic pain has been facilitated by widespread of neuro-imaging methods that helped to explore a link between functional changes in neuronal networks and chronic pain. The evidence gained over the past two decades suggests that i) patients with certain chronic pain syndromes develop changes in the excitability and/or somatotopic organization within certain brain areas (e.g. in the motor or somatosensory cortex, thalamus and others) (1-7) normalization/modulation of such changes can be paralleled by pain relief (8-13).

Indeed, an application of invasive- or non- invasive brain stimulation in selected populations with chronic pain of neuropathic origin (e.g. central pain due to thalamic infarction, spinal cord injury, multiple sclerosis, complex regional pain syndrome, fibromyalgia) resulted in significant pain relief (14-25) suggesting a promising analgesic potential of such a neuromodulatory-treatment paradigm.

The invasive approach is represented by two main techniques, Deep Brain Stimulation (DBS), and epidural Motor Cortex Stimulation (MCS). DBS is an electrical stimulation performed after stereotactic implantation of thin stick leads into subcortical areas like e. g. thalamus or basal ganglia. MCS (see Figure 1) is an electrical stimulation of the precentral gyrus using epidural surgical leads and subthreshold stimulation.

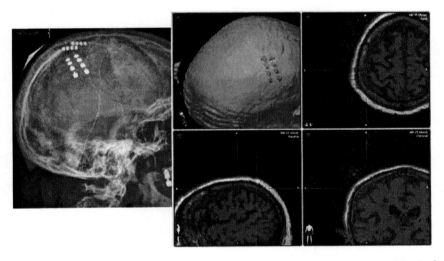

Figure 1. An example of Invasive Epidural Motor Cortex Stimulation (MCS). Left: Lateral x-ray of the skull documenting the position of the implanted paddle leads. Right: matching of postoperative ct-scan and preoperative MRI-3D- neuronavigation data with inserted position of the leads over the pre- and postcentral gyrus. (Courtesy of Dr. Rasche).

Non-invasive brain stimulation approaches include two main techniques, Transcranial Magnetic Stimulation (TMS) and Transcranial Direct Current Stimulation (tDCS). TMS is based on the principle of electromagnetic induction to focus induced currents in the brain. TDCS (see Figure 2) uses low intensity direct current penetrating through the scalp to the brain, influencing neuronal excitability and modulating the firing rates of individual neurons.

In this chapter, we review and discuss evidence on the use of both invasive- and non-invasive brain stimulation techniques for the treatment of neuropathic facial pain.

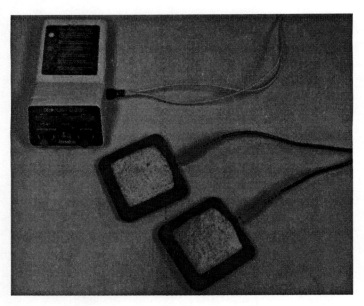

Figure 2. An example of device for the non-invasive Transcranial Direct Current Stimulation (tDCS). TDCS uses low intensity direct current penetrating through the scalp to the brain, influencing neuronal excitability and modulating the firing rates of individual neurons. (Courtesy of Drs. Knotkova and Cruciani).

Neuropathic facial pain

Neuropathic facial pain is a debilitating condition characterized by burning, stabbing pain and disesthetic sensations in the distribution of the trigeminal nerve. Neuropathic facial pain arises due to various causes and presents with a variety of symptoms. As a result, numerous classification-systems exist and facial-pain terminology is not unified. Although it is not directly stated, numerous studies as reviewed in this article (see below) refer to facial-pain terminology that corresponds to a high degree with the classification system by Burchiel (26) that distinguishes seven diagnostic entities according to the cause of damage to the trigeminal nerve:

Brain Stimulation for the treatment of neuropathic facial pain   135

- *Trigeminal neuralgia, type 1,* (TN1): facial pain of spontaneous onset with predominantly episodic pain.
- *Trigeminal neuralgia, type 2,* (TN2): facial pain of spontaneous onset with predominantly constant pain.
- *Symptomatic trigeminal neuralgia,* (STN): pain resulting from disturbance of trigeminal nerve by a demyelinating plaque in the central pathway of the trigeminal nerve due to multiple sclerosis.
- *Trigeminal neuropathic pain,* (TNP): facial pain resulting from unintentional injury to the trigeminal system from facial trauma, oral surgery, ear, nose and throat (ENT) surgery, root injury from posterior fossa or skull base surgery, stroke, etc.
- *Trigeminal deafferentation pain,* (TDP): facial pain in a region of trigeminal numbness resulting from intentional injury to the trigeminal system from neurectomy, gangliolysis, rhizotomy, nucleotomy, tractotomy, or other neuroablative procedures.
- *Postherpetic neuralgia,* (PHN): pain resulting from trigeminal Herpes zoster (shingles) outbreak in the trigeminal distribution. The pain is often described as constant, intense, and unbearable, frequently with presence of allodynia.
- *Atypical facial pain,* (AFP): pain having a substantial psychological component or being psychological rather than of physiological origin.

Successful treatment of neuropathic facial pain is of high importance because it can cause severe impairment of patient's daily functioning and substantially decrease quality of patients' life. There is a wide spectrum of pharmacological agents that can be used for pain management of neuropathic facial pain, for example antidepressants, anticonvulsants, and other drugs like muscle relaxants and steroids, and in selected cases also opioids. However, many patients experience unbearable drug-induced side effects and remain with excruciating pain and severe impairment of function despite multiple treatment cycles with a variety and combinations of the agents listed above. In those patients, non-pharmacological treatment strategies, including brain stimulation techniques, may represent a promising option to explore. Brain stimulation techniques target central neuroplastic functional changes in the brain (e.g. pathological alterations in activity in the somatosensory cortex, motor cortex or thalamus), which have been observed in numerous studies in patients with chronic pain (1-5,27). Indeed, a recent study by DaSilva and colleagues (28) confirmed the existence of functional (as well as structural) cortical changes in patients with facial neuropathic pain, supporting the rationale for the use of brain stimulation in facial neuropathic pain, and indicating that this patient-population may benefit from brain-stimulation treatment strategies.

Invasive brain stimulation

Deep Brain Stimulation (DBS)

The experience with DBS for the management of trigeminal neuropathic pain is limited (29-33) (see Table 1).

In 1997, Kumar and colleagues (29) evaluated their experience with the DBS thalamic implantation targeting nucleus ventralis posterior medialis (VPM) in patients with various diagnoses (total n=68), including four patients with trigeminal neuropathy. All four patients with the neuropathic facial pain experienced an excellent pain relief during entire follow up period that ranged between 12 and 28 months. Similarly, in a case-observation by Green and colleagues (30), a patient with a 10-year history of post-herpetic trigeminal neuralgia who underwent a successful treatment with DBS targeting the region of periventricular grey area (PVG) contralateral to the site of pain, and ventral posterior lateral thalamic nucleus (VPL) experienced substantial pain relief. Pain intensity decreased from 6.9/10 prior the procedure to 0-1/10 (0= no pain, 10= severe/maximum pain) after the lead implant, and at the last follow-up six months later, the patient remained pain free.

Rasche and colleagues (31) within a series of 56 patients with various chronic neuropathic pain syndromes, observed pain reduction of > 25% up to 100% by DBS that combined stimulation of VPM and PVG in 4/6 patients with dysesthesia dolorosa in trigeminal nerve region.

Cordella and colleagues (33) performed DBS in five patients for the treatment of trigeminal neuralgia due to multiple sclerosis (i.e. Symptomatic Trigeminal Neuralgia in the classification system by Burchiel (26) with a specific aim to assess the efficacy of the DBS on the paroxysmal ophthalmic pain.

Table 1. Studies and Case-observations Using Deep Brain Stimulation (DBS) in Patients with Neuropathic Facial Pain

Authors	Sample Size (facial/total n)	Design	Parameters of Stimulation					Side Effects
			Location	Freq	Voltage, Pulse Width	Stimulation		
Kumar et al., 1997[29]	4/68	Case Series	Nucleus ventralis posterior medialis	50 – 100 Hz	2 – 8 V, 0.2 – 0.8ms	ON for 60 sec, OFF for 10 min		Several mild side effects, non life-threatening.
Green et al., 2002[30]	1/1	Case Report	Ventral posterior lateral thalamic nucleus	250 Hz	1.5 – 2.5 V, 210ms	Intermittent		None reported.
Rasche et al., 2006[31]	6/56	Open label	Nucleus ventralis posterior medialis, periventricular grey	40-90	1-3.5 V	Cyclic and/or continuous		None reported
Broggi et al., 2007[32]	3/16	Case Series	Posterior nucleus of the hypothalamus	180 Hz	$1 - 3$ V, 60µs	Continuous		None reported.
Cordella et al., 2009[33]	5/5	Open Label	Posterior nucleus of the hypothalamus	180 Hz	$1 - 2$V, 60ms	Continuous		None reported.

Table 2. Studies and Case-observations Using Motor Cortex Stimulation (MCS) in Patients with Neuropathic Facial Pain

Authors	Sample Size (facial/ total n)	Design	Parameters for Stimulation					Side Effects
			Leads	Freq	Voltage, Pulse Width	Stimulation		
Meyerson et al., 1993[36]	5/10	Open label	1 quadripolar	50 Hz	0.6 to 0.8ms	20 -30 mins sessions, 1-6 sessions/day		Short-lasting generalized seizures
Herregodts et al., 1995[37]	7/7	Open label	1 quadripolar	50-75 Hz	4 to 8V, 0.8ms	Intermittent 1 hr six times/day		None reported.
Ebel et al., 1996[38]	7/7	Open label	1 quadripolar	60-130 Hz	3.5 to 8.5V, 180-350µs	Continuous, 3 hrs OFF, 20-30 mins ON		1 subject developed a seizure
Nguyen et al., 2000[39]	12/32	Open label	1 quadripolar	40 Hz	2.1V, 82.5µs	Continuous 3 hrs ON, 3 hrs OFF for 12 hrs per day		Subcutaneous infection (1); dehiscence of the scar (1); headache (3); asymptomatic epidural hematoma (1);
Rainov and Heidecke, 2003[40]	2/2	Open label	1 quadripolar	100 Hz	5-8.5 V, 300-400ms	Intermittent 1 hr ON, 1 hr OFF, total 6-9 hrs delivered per day		A single episode of epileptic seizure.
Brown and Pilitsis, 2005[41]	10/10	Open label	1 four array	40 Hz	2 to 8V, 90 to 240µs	Info not provided		Postoperative wound infection (1 patient)

Authors	Sample Size (facial/ total n)	Design	Parameters for Stimulation					Side Effects
			Leads	Freq	Voltage, Pulse Width	Stimulation		
Rasche et al., 2006[42]	10/17	Double-Blinded with sham stimulation	1 or 2 quadripolar	5-100Hz	2.5 to 10V, 210-360µs	Intermittent early after implantation From 3x 0.5hr to 1hr ON 0.5 hr OFF; then continuous		Intraoperative seizure (7 patients); wound infection (1 patient); speech arrest for three months with complete resolution (1 patient);
Lefaucheur et al., 2009[43]	6/16	Crossover trial was performed between 1 and 3 months postoperative, followed by an open phase	1 quadripolar	40Hz	2V, 60µs	Continuous		None reported.
Anderson et al, 2009[44]	1	Case Report	1 quadripolar	5 Hz	2mA, 250µs	Intermittent 36 hrs ON, 12 hrs OFF during the trial. No info		None reported.
Fontaine et al, 2009[45]	1	Case Report	1 quadipolar	40Hz	3V, 210µs	Not stated		None reported.
Esfahani et al, 2010[46]	3/3	Case Series	5-6-5	43.3 ± 5.8 Hz	1.6 ± 1.4 V	Not stated.		Subjects reported minor facial spasms, headaches and facial swelling.

In patients with multiple sclerosis, the ophthalmic branch of trigeminal nerve is frequently disturbed and the risks carried by conventional neurosurgical ablative procedures are high and include major adverse effects such as corneal reflex impairment and keratitis. The patients (n=5) underwent implantation of DBS leads into the hypothalamic posterior nucleus. Follow-up period ranged between 11 months and 4 years; the evaluation of outcomes was done on daily basis for the first two weeks, then every three months. All five patients reported immediate pain relief, followed by a protracted period of long-term pain control, a reduced need for analgesic medication, and improved quality of life. Pain relief specific to ophthalmic branch of trigeminal nerve (i.e. the pain relief which was primarily targeted by the procedure) sustained for the entire follow up period in all five patients. Pain relief related to second and/or third trigeminal branch was recurrent after 11-28 months. No side effects or morbidity of the procedure was reported.

Broggy and colleagues (32) reported results of DBS of posterior thalamus in a mixed sample of patients, including three patients with atypical facial pain (besides 17 headache patients; total n=20). Although the headache patients benefited form the continuous DBS stimulation, DBS had no effect in the atypical-facial-pain patients.

Epidural motor cortex stimulation (MCS)

There is more experience with MCS than with DBS for the treatment of facial pain of neuropathic origin. It is estimated (34,35) that about 150 patients with TNP were treated and implanted with MCS worldwide.

We have identified 11 reports that utilized MCS to treat neuropathic facial pain (36-46) (see Table 2). Meyerson and colleagues (36) were the first to report experience with MCS in patients with trigeminal neuropathic pain (n=5) following surgery in the trigeminal territory. All these subjects presented with pain, abnormalities of facial sensation dominated by dysaesthesia or allodynia to mechanical stimuli and hyperalgesia to pin prick. MCS in all five patients with TNP resulted in substantial pain relief >50% (pain relief in two of them reached >75%). During the testing phase most patients had one or two short-lasting generalizes seizures, but no seizures occurred after permanent implantation. Two patients experienced local painful sensation at the craniotomy or site of the implanted lead. One patient developed epidural hematoma leading to aphasia. At the time of the last follow up, the patient still presented with slight form of dysphasia. Re-operation at the site of the

Brain Stimulation for the treatment of neuropathic facial pain 141

connection located behind the ear, due to possible ulceration, was necessary in two patients.

In the study by Herregodts and colleagues (37) MCS was performed in seven patients (1 trigeminal neuralgia, 4 trigeminal neuropathic pain due to damaged trigeminal nerve after surgery, 1 pain in the face and upper extremity due to post-stroke central pain syndrome; 1 patient had post-stroke pain in upper body but not in face). Follow up period ranged between 4 and 22 months. Full pain relief was achieved in 1 patient with TNP; pain relief > 50% was reported in five of seven patients. One patient (post-stroke pain in upper body) did not respond to MCS at all, and one patient with TNP experienced minor temporary pain relief (20% to 0 in 6 weeks).

Ebel and colleagues (38) reported a case series of 7 patients with severe TNP (n=6) and postherpetic neuralgia (n=1) involving the first and second division of trigeminal nerve. The length of pain history ranged between 1 and 21 years. In all but one case, the impulse generator was implanted after a successful period of test stimulation. Stimulation parameters (see table 2) were individually adjusted so that they were close to the motor threshold. The follow up period ranged from 6 months up to 2 years. In three patients (all with TNP) the stimulation resulted in excellent long-term pain relief (100% n=2, 80-100% n=1) at the last follow up. In two patients (1 postherpetic neuralgia, 1 TNP) pain relief ranged between 80%-40%, declining over time. In one patient (TNP), frequency of pain episodes decreased, but pain-intensity change was minimal. Side effects were observed in one patient who developed a prolonged focal seizure with a postictal speech arrest during test stimulation; the permanent impulse generator was not implanted in this patient.

Nguyen and colleagues (39) performed MCS in 32 patients (18 M, 14 F) with neuropathic pain. Of those, 12 patients had TNP secondary to thermal rhizotomy, ENT operation, postoperative brainstem lesion or skull base trauma. Pain history ranged between 4-14 years. Follow up period after lead implantation ranged between 3 and 50 months. Results showed that nine of the twelve patients with TNP experienced good or satisfactory pain relief (8 pt and 1 pt respectively). Several adverse events were noted in the study: subcutaneous infection (1 patient), partial dehiscence of the stimulator pocket scar (1 patient), headache (3 patients), asymptomatic epidural hematoma (1 patient). No episodes of epilepsy were noted.

Rainov and Heidecke (40) reported results of MCS in two cases with facial pain due to trigeminal neuralgia and surgical trauma to the glossopharyngeal nerve, respectively. Follow up period was 72 and 69 months.

Pain decreased from 7/10 to mean 3/10 and from 8/10 to mean 2/10 respectively. One single episode of epilepsy was noted.

Brown and Philitsis (41) published findings form a prospective study of 10 patients with central- and peripheral neuropathic facial pain. Four patients had trigeminal neuropathic pain following trigeminal nerve root injury, two patients had trigeminal postherpetic neuralgia, two patients had facial pain and history of thalamic or brainstem infarction and in two patients the cause was unknown. Pain history ranged between 1 and 12 years and follow up period between 3 and 24 months. As result of MCS, eight patients experienced pain relief > 50% during a testing phase and in these patients the neurostimulator was implanted. At the follow up, pain relief still remained > 50%. Besides pain relief, three patients experienced improved facial sensory discrimination and motor strength, and one patient had improved dysarthria. In each of these patients, the improvements were positively correlated with active or non-active MCS. No seizures were observed. Due to postoperative wound infection removal and later re-implantation of the lead and pulse generator was necessary in one patient.

Rasche and colleagues (42) retrospectively evaluated a group of neuropathic pain patients with follow up period up to 10 years (mean 3.6 years) to assess MCS for long-term relief of neuropathic pain. Seventeen patients (10 with TNP; 7 with post-stroke pain) and pain history ranging between 2-12 years were evaluated. All patients underwent a test trial during which double-blind testing was conducted. Double-blind testing identified 6 non-responders. Among responders, 5 of 10 patients with TNP (and 3 of 7 with post-stroke pain) had pain reduction ≥50% at the time of last follow up. Intra-operative seizures were observed in 7 patients, wound infection in 1 patient, and 1 patient developed speech arrest for three months, with complete resolution. Lefaucheur and colleagues (43) reported the first randomized controlled trial evaluating chronic MCS in the treatment of refractory peripheral neuropathic pain. The sample of 16 patients consisted of six patients with facial pain (four trigeminal neuralgia, one trigeminal post herpetic neuralgia, one atypical orofacial pain secondary to dental extraction). The remaining 10 subjects had brachial plexus lesion [4], neurofibromatosis [3], limb amputation [2], nerve trunk transaction in lower limb [1]. A quadripolar lead was implanted for epidural MCS. A randomized cross-over trial was performed between 1 and 3 months postoperative, during which the stimulator was alternatively switched ON and OFF for 1 month, followed by an open phase during which the stimulator was ON in all patients. Significant difference between ON vs OFF stimulation were found in pain-rating index as well as sensory sub-score as both measured by McGill Pain Questionnaire. Clinical follow up period was up to one year. Anderson and colleagues (44) implemented MCS in a patient with neuropathic facial pain that included elements of trigeminal neuralgia, glossopharyngeal neuralgia and dysphagia. After failing pharmacological and surgical decompressive treatments, the patient underwent a successful MCS trial followed by implantation of a neurostimulation device. During the MCS trial, pain decreased from VAS 10 to 7; after the implantation, pain increased again, but adjustment of stimulation parameters resulted in satisfactory pain relief as well as substantial improvement in swallowing, absence of gagging sensation and a reduction in episodes of nausea and vomiting. At 2 years, MCS generator was replaced and patient continued to experience benefits from MCS. Improvement of symptoms, namely the improvement of dysphagia had profound positive impact on the patient's functional status. Fontaine and colleagues (45) reported a case in which MCS improved TNP and restored tactile and thermal sensory loss. The patient developed intractable pain after trauma of the supraorbital branch of the trigeminal nerve, associated with tactile and thermal sensory loss in the painful area. One month after MCS implantation, pain intensity decreased from NRS 80/100 to 20/100, paralleled with sensory-discrimination improvement. Two months after MCS implant, normalization of thermal-detection thresholds was noted. Subdural placement of a surgical lead over the precentral gyrus was performed by Esfahani and colleagues (46) in three patients with intractable facial pain (deafferentation pain following rhizotomy, secondary to meningioma surgery and postherpetic neuralgia). In these three patients pain reduction of more than 50% by active MCS was achieved. As noted by Levy and colleagues (35) in a recent review on MCS and DBS for pain control, MCS is favoured for more anatomically localized pain syndromes like TNP, post-stroke pain or brachial plexus avulsion, while DBS is considerable also in mixed (neuropathic and nociceptive) pain syndromes.

Non-invasive brain stimulation techniques

Repetitive transcranial magnetic stimulation (rTMS)

Although no rTMS studies targeted exclusively facial-pain population, various rTMS trials in neuropathic pain (47-55) (see Table 3) included patients with neuropathic facial pain as a sub-population of study samples (total n=231, neuropathic facial pain n=74).

The main purpose of these trials was to explore various rTMS parameters, target groups and designs of rTMS in order to maximize its analgesic potential as non-invasive and safer variant to invasive brain stimulation techniques.

A double-blind sham-controlled study by Lefaucheur and colleagues (47) involving seven patients with chronic treatment-resistant trigeminal neuropathy patients and seven patients central pain due to thalamic stroke who were registered candidates for invasive MCS implant, was the first one showing that high frequency (20 Hz) rTMS delivered over the motor cortex in patients with treatment resistant neuropathic pain can overlast the time of stimulation, though the duration of the effect was neither permanent nor long-lasting. In this study, a single session of real high-frequency rTMS over the motor cortex and a single session of sham were delivered in a three-week interval in the double-blind manner. In the trigeminal neuropathy group, individual results showed a significant pain relief (>30%) in 4 of 7 patients, and the same results were observed also in the post-stroke group. The overall evaluation showed statistically significant decrease in pain intensity after real rTMS but not sham for days 1 to 8 after the stimulation; from day 9 to 12 the difference between results from sham vs real rTMS was not significant. Although the pain-relief induced by high frequency rTMS in this study was short-lasting, the findings provided initial evidence for further explorations of stimulation-parameters to optimize rTMS analgesic effects. Findings from later studies (49,51) performed in patients with various types of neuropathic pain (total n=96), including neuropathic facial pain (n=30), suggested that pain origin, site of pain and somatotopic area to which the stimulation is targeted are significant variables determining the analgesic outcomes of the stimulation. As for origin of pain, rTMS was significantly less effective in patients with pain due to brainstem stroke as compared with pain due to trigeminal nerve lesion, spinal cord- or brachial plexus lesion. For pain-site, facial pain yielded better response to the stimulation than pain in upper or lower limb. Regarding somatotopic area targeted by the stimulation, analgesic effects were better when the stimulation was applied to the area adjacent to the cortical representation of the painful zone than to the motor cortical area corresponding to the painful zone itself. For example, patients with facial pain experienced better pain relief when the stimulation targeted cortical M1 representation of hand which is a representation adjacent to M1 somatotopic representation of face.

Table 3. Studies and Case-observations Using Repetitive Transcranial Magnetic Stimulation (rTMS) in Patients with Neuropathic Facial Pain

Authors	Sample Size (facial/ total n)	Design	Parameters for Stimulation					Side Effects
			Number of sessions	Trains of stimulation	Freq	Intensity (% of Motor Threshold)		
Lefaucheur et al., 2001[47]	7/14	Randomized, blinded study	1 session	20 trains of 5 second stimulations	10 Hz	80%		None reported.
Rollnik et al., 2002[48]	1/12	Randomized, blinded study	1 session	20 trains of 2 second stimulations	20 Hz	80%		None reported.
Lefaucheur et al., 2004[49]	12/60	Randomized, blinded study	1 session	20 trains of 5 second stimulations	10 Hz	80%		None reported.
Khedr et al., 2005[50]	24/48	Randomized, blinded study	5 sessions	10 trains of 10 second stimulations	20 Hz	80%		None reported.
Lefaucheur et al., 2006[51]	18/36	Open label	2 sessions	20 trains of 10 second stimulations	10 Hz	90%		None reported.
Hirayama et al., 2006[52]	3/20	Open label	4 sessions	20 trains of 10 second stimulations	5 Hz	90%		None reported.
André-Obadia et al., 2006[53]	1/12	Double-blind, randomized	3 sessions	20 trains of 80 stimulations	1 or 20 Hz	90%		None reported.
André-Obadia et al., 2008[54]	7/28	Double-blind, randomized, with cross-over	2 session	20 trains of 80 stimulations	20 Hz	90%		None reported.
Zaghi et al., 2009[55]	1/1	Longitudinal (1 yr) case observation	35 sessions in four treatment blocks (10, 10, 5, 10)	30 trains of 4 second stimulations	10 Hz	Info not provided		Occasional mild head and neckaches.

Similarly, patients with neuropathic pain localized in hand or arm experienced better results when the stimulation targeted M1 area corresponding with cortical representation of face (51). Further studies (52-54) in patients with various types of neuropathic pain (total n=60), including neuropathic facial pain (n=11) suggested better analgesic- as well as predictive properties of high frequency rTMS as compared to low frequency rTMS or sham. For example, a double-blind study by Andre-Obadia and colleagues (53) compared analgesic effect of 1Hz and 20 Hz rTMS stimulation frequencies against sham, and determined correlation between rTMS and MCS efficacy in order to assess predictive value of rTMS for efficacy of MCS implants. Fourteen patients with chronic treatment-resistant neuropathic pain (trigeminal-, central post-stroke-, and peripheral brachial plexus neuropathic pain), who were referred for invasive MCS, received three double-blind sessions (1 Hz rTMS, 20 Hz rTMS and sham) in random order with 2-week interval between sessions. Pain intensity ratings six days after each session were compared to the baseline as well as correlated with those obtained from subsequently applied invasive MCS. Finings indicated that 1 Hz rTMS yielded poorest analgesic results, decreasing pain ratings only immediately after- but not one week after the stimulation, and being pro-algesic in some patients. On contrary, decrease of pain intensity by 20 Hz rTMS was still present one week after the stimulation and only 20 Hz rTMS but not sham or 1 Hz rTMS predicted the efficacy of subsequent MCS.

To explore possible prolongation of analgesic effect of 20 Hz rTMS, Khedr and colleagues (50) applied five daily sessions (instead of a single session as reported in previous studies) of high frequency (20 Hz) rTMS in 24 patients with trigeminal neuralgia and 24 patients with post-stroke pain syndrome. In this study, the set of five real 20 Hz rTMS sessions lead to significantly better pain-improvement than sham and the effect was evident even at the two-week follow-up after the treatment. Average pain relief of 45% was reported among TN participants in the active rTMS group, with 79% of participants acknowledging significant pain relief persisting for the follow-up period of two weeks, indicating that repeated rTMS sessions can produce longer-lasting pain relief. Further exploring repeated use of rTMS, Zahni and colleagues (55) aimed to determine whether rTMS could indeed be used longitudinally for pain management in clinical settings. A patient with refractory trigeminal neuralgia received high frequency (10 Hz) rTMS over the motor cortex in four treatment periods over one year. The treatment periods consisted of 10, 10, 5 and 10 rTMS sessions respectively. The interval between the treatment period was 4 months, 2 weeks, 3 months and 1 month respectively. The primary outcome was self-reported overall daily pain intensity. The results showed that although individual treatment periods could result in significant and meaningful pain relief, the observed effects were persistent to about maximum of four weeks after the end of stimulation period. This longitudinal case-observation however demonstrated that repeated long term application of rTMS is safe and would be beneficial, though costly therapy. This latter finding indirectly points to another non-invasive modulatory technique, transcranial direct current stimulation (tDCS).

Transcranial direct current stimulation

TDCS has been shown to be less expensive, easy to implement, and portable alternative to rTMS. TDCS has been shown to alleviate neuropathic pain in patients with various chronic pain syndromes. Although up to date there are no findings from randomized sham-controlled studies in patients with neuropathic facial pain yet, open-label tDCS was successfully applied in two clinical cases of patients with trigeminal neuralgia and neuropathic facial pain due to surgical disturbance of trigeminal nerve respectively (56). In both cases, 5 sessions of tDCS applied on five consecutive days resulted in decrease of pain scores > 50% and lead to decrease of consumption of "as needed" pain-medication used to manage break through pain. Although these very preliminary findings indicate clinical usefulness of tDCS in the treatment of neuropathic pain, sham-controlled studies in larger samples are warranted.

Conclusions

In patients with neuropathic facial pain, recent evidence (28) confirmed the existence of pain-driven functional neuroplastic changes in the brain, further supporting the rationale for the use of brain stimulation in facial neuropathic pain and corroborating empirical evidence that this patient-population may benefit from brain-stimulation treatment-strategies.

The results from prospective controlled studies as well as clinical case reports that included patients with neuropathic facial pain indicate that both invasive- and non-invasive brain stimulation can significantly alleviate neuropathic facial pain. The group of patients treated with invasive brain-stimulation techniques were mainly patients with highly-disabling, intractable pain resistant to a wide spectrum of other treatment options. It has been recognized that due to the nature of potential side-effects and higher risk for the patient, the invasive brain stimulation should be reserved for carefully selected patients as the last-resort treatment. Although, when successfully applied, the invasive approach enables to apply the stimulation in a long-term mode (several hours ON, several hours OFF for months or even years) and thus providing long-term pain relief.

Non-invasive rTMS stimulation in populations with neuropathic pain, including patients with neuropathic facial pain, indicated that rTMS of higher frequencies can significantly alleviate neuropathic facial pain. Non-invasive brain stimulation mainly serves patients who want to explore non-pharmacological treatment-options, i.e. patients whose facial pain does not respond to conventional pharmacological treatment, or when medication (for medical or other reasons) can not be used or optimized to provide sufficient pain relief. Non-invasive rTMS in facial pain patients has also been preliminary explored as a predictor for efficacy of invasive MCS implants. Although the duration of the rTMS analgesic effect in existing protocols is limited to maximum of several weeks, preliminary findings from a longitudinal case-observation of patient with trigeminal neuralgia indicated clinical benefits from repeated rTMS treatments, justifying further studies exploring long-term pain control by rTMS as well as by tDCS in populations with neuropathic facial pain.

References

[1] Flor H, Braun C, Elbert T, Birbaumer N. Extensive reorganization of primary somatosensory cortex in chronic back pain patients. Neurosci Lett 1997;224:5-8.

[2] Flor H. The functional organization of the brain in chronic pain. In: Sandkühler J, Bromm B, Gebhart GF, eds. Progress in brain research, Vol 129. Amsterdam: Elsevier, 2000:313-22.

[3] Maihöfner C, Handwerker HO, Neundorfer B, Birklein F. Patterns of cortical reorganization in complex regional pain syndrome. Neurology 2003;61:1717-25.

[4] Tinazzi M, Valeriani M, Moretto G, Rosso T, Nicolato A, Fiaschi A, Aglioti SM. Plastic interactions between hand and face cortical representations in patients with trigeminal neuralgia: a somatosensory-evoked potentials study. Neurosci 2004;127:769-76.

[5] Eisenberg E, Chystiakov AV, Yudashkin M, Kaplan B, Hafner H, Feinsod M. Evidence for cortical hyperexcitability of the affected limb representation area in CRPS: a psychophysical and transcranial magnetic stimulation study. Pain 2005;113:99-105.

Brain Stimulation for the treatment of neuropathic facial pain 149

[6] Chen R, Cohen LG, Hallett M. Nervous system reorganization following injury. Neuroscience 2002;111:761-73.

[7] Cohen LG, Bandinelli S, Findley TW, Hallett M. Motor reorganization after upper limb amputation in man. Brain 1991;114:615-27.

[8] Flor H. The modification of cortical reorganization and chronic pain by sensory feedback. Appl Psychophysiol Biofeedback 2002;27:215-27.

[9] Flor H. Cortical reorganization and chronic pain: implications for rehabilitation. J Rehabil Med 2003;41:66-72.

[10] Maihöfner CCA, Handwerker HO, Neundorfer B, Birklein F. Cortical reorganization during recovery from complex regional pain syndrome. Neurology 2004;63:693-701.

[11] Passard A, Attal N, Benadhira R, Brasseur L, Saba G, Sichere P, et al. Effects of unilateral repetitive transcranial magnetic stimulation of the motor cortex on chronic widespread pain in fibromyalgia. Brain 2007;130:2661-70.

[12] Pleger B, Tegenthoff M, Ragert P, Forster AF, Dinse H, Nicolas PV, Maier C. Sensorimotor returning in complex regional pain syndrome parallels pain reduction. Ann Neurol 2005;57:425-29.

[13] Brown JA, Barbaro NM. Motor cortex stimulation for central and neuropathic pain: current status. Pain 2003;104:431-35.

[14] Pleger B, Janssen F, Schwenkreis P, Volker B, Maier C, Tegenthoff M. Repetitive transcranial magnetic stimulation of the motor cortex attenuates pain perception in complex regional pain syndrome type I. Neurosci Lett 2004;356:87-90.

[15] Rollnik JD, Wustefeld S, Dauper M, Karst M, Fink M, Kossev A, Dengler R. Repetitive transcranial magnetic stimulation for the treatment of chronic pain – a pilot study. Eur Neurol 2002;48:6-10.

[16] Smania N, Corato E, Fiaschi A, Pietropoli P, Aglioti SM, Tinazzi M. Repetitive magnetic stimulation: a novel therapeutic approach for myofascial pain syndrome. J Neurol 2005;252:307-14.

[17] Topper R, Foltys H, Meister IG, Sparing R, Boroojerdi B. Repetitive transcranial magnetic stimulation of the parietal cortex transiently ameliorates phantom limb pain-like syndrome. Clin Neurophysiol 2003;114:1521-30.

[18] Canavero S, Bonicalzi V, Dotta M, Vighetti S, Asteggiano G, Cocito D. Transcranial magnetic cortical stimulation relieves central pain. Stereotact Funct Neurosurg 2002;78:192-96.

[19] Khedr EM, Kotb H, Kamel NF, Ahmed MA, Sadek R, Rothwell JC. Longlasting antalgic effects of daily sessions of repetitive transcranial magnetic stimulation in central and peripheral neuropathic pain. J Neurol Neurosurg Psychiatry 2005;76:833-38.

[20] Fregni F, Gimenes R, Valle AS, Ferreira MJ, Rocha RR, Natalle L, et al. A randomized,sham-controlled, proof of principle study of transcranial direct current stimulation for the treatment of pain in fibromyalgia. Arthritis Rheum 2006; 54(12):3988-98.

[21] Fregni F, Boggio PS, Lima MC, Ferreira MJ, Wagner T, Rigonatti SP, et al. A sham-controlled, phase II trial of transcranial direct current stimulation for the treatment of central pain in traumatic spinal cord injury. Pain 2006;122(1-2):197-209.

150 Helena Knotkova, Arash Nafissi, Eliah Soto et al.

[22] Andre-Obadia N, Peyron R, Mertens P, Mauguiere F, Laurent B,Garcia-Larea L. Transcranial magnetic stimulation for pain control. Double-blind study of different frequencies against placebo, and correlation with motor cortex stimulation efficacy. Clin Neurophysiol 2006;117:1536-44.

[23] Knotkova H, Esteban S, Sibirceva U, Das D, Cruciani RA. Non-invasive brain stimulation therapy for the management of cmplex regional pain síndrome (CRPS). In: Knotkova H, Cruciani RA, Merrick J, eds.: Pain. Brain stimulation in the treatment of pain. New York: Nova Science, 2010:155-68.

[24] Knotkova H, Cruciani RA. Non-invasive transcranial direct current stimulation for the study and treatment of neuropathic pain. In: Szallaszi A, ed. Methods in molecular biology: Pain and anesthesia. New York: Humana Press, Springer, 2010:505-17.

[25] Antal A, Terney D, Kühnl S, Paulus W. Anodal transcranial direct current stimulation of the motor cortex ameliorates chronic pain and reduces short intracortical inhibition. J Pain Symptom Manage 2010;39(5):890-903.

[26] Burchiel KJ. A new classification for facial pain. Neurosurgery 2003;53(5):1164-7.

[27] Pascual-Leone A, Peris M, Tormos JM, Pascual-leone Pascual A, Catala MD. Reorganization of human cortical motor output maps following traumatic forearm amputation. NeuroReport 1996;7:2068-70.

[28] DaSilva AF, Becerra L, Pendse G, Chizh B, Tully S, Borsook D. Colocalized structural and functional changes in the cortex of patients with trigeminal neuropathic pain. PLoS One 2008;3(10):e3396.

[29] Kumar K, Toth C, Nath RK. Deep brain stimulation for intractable pain: a 15-year experience. Neurosurgery 1997;4:736-47.

[30] Green AL, Nandi D, Armstrong G, Carter H, Aziz T. Post-herpetic trigeminal neuralgia treated with deep brain stimulation. J Clin Neurosci 2003;4:512-14.

[31] Rasche D, Rinaldi PC, Young RF, Tronnier VM. Deep brain stimulation for the treatment of various chronic pain syndromes. Neurosurg Focus 2006;21(6):E8.

[32] Broggi G, Franzini A, Leone M, Bussone G. Update on neurosurgical treatment of chronic trigeminal autonomic cephalalgias and atypical facial pain with deep brain stimulation of posterior hypothalamus: Results and comments. Neurol Sci 2007;(Suppl 2):S138-45.

[33] Cordella R, Franzini A, La Mantia L, Marras C, Erbetta A, Broggi G. Hypothalamic stimulation for trigeminal neuralgia in multiple sclerosis patients: efficacy on the paroxysmal ophthalmic pain. Mult Scler 2009;11:1322-8.

[34] Rasche D, Tronnier VM. Extradural cortical stimulation for peripheral (including trigeminal) neuropathic pain. In: Canavero S, ed. Textbook of therapeutic cortical stimulation. New York: Nova Science, 2009.

[35] Levy R, Deer TR, Henderson J. Intracranial neurostimulation for pain control: a review. Pain Physician 2010;13:157-65.

[36] Meyerson B, Lindblom U, Linderoth B, Lind G, Herregodts P. Motor cortex stimulation as treatment of trigeminal neuropathic pain. Acta Neurochir Suppl 1993;58:150-3.

Brain Stimulation for the treatment of neuropathic facial pain 151

[37] Herregodts P, Stadnik T, De Ridder F, D'Haens J. Cortical stimulation of central neuropathic pain:3-D surface MRI for easy determination of the motor cortex. Acta Neurochir Suppl 1995;64:132-5.

[38] Ebel H, Rust D, Tronnier V, Böker D, Kunze S. Chronic precentral stimulation in trigeminal neuropathic pain. Acta Neurochir 1996;138:1300-6.

[39] Nguyen J, Lefaucher J, Le Guerinel C, Eizenbaum J, Nakano N, Carpentier A, et al. Motor cortex stimulation in the treatment of central and neuropathic pain. Arch Med Res 2000;31:263-5.

[40] Rainov N, Heidecke V. Motor cortex stimulation for neuropathic facial pain. Neurol Res 2003;25:157-61.

[41] Brown J, Pilitsis J. Motor cortex stimulation for central and neuropathic facial pain: A prospective study of 10 patients and observation of enhanced sensory and motor function during stimulation. Neurosurgery 2005;56:290-7.

[42] Rasche D, Ruppolt M, Stippich C, Unterberg A, Tronnier V. Motor cortex stimulation for long-term relief of chronic neuropathic pain: A 10 year experience. Pain 2006;121:43-52.

[43] Lefaucheur J, Drouot X, Cunin P, Bruckert R, Lepetit H, Créange A, et al. Motor cortex stimulation for the treatment of refractory peripheral neuropathic pain. Brain 2009;132:1463-71.

[44] Anderson W, Kiyofuji S, Conway J, Busch C, North R, Garonzik I. Dysphagia and neuropathic facial pain treated with motor cortex stimulation: Case report. Neurosurgery 2009;65:E626.

[45] Fontaine D, Bruneto J, El Fakir H, Paquis P, Lanteri-Minet M. Short-term restoration of facial sensory loss by motor cortex stimulation in peripheral post-traumatic neuropathic pain. J Headache Pain 2009;10:203-6.

[46] Esfahani DR, Pisansky MT, Dafer RM, Anderson DE. Motor cortex stimulation: functional magnetic resonance imaging – localized treatment for three sources of intractable facial pain. J Neurosurg 2010, DOI: 10.3171/2010.5.JNS091696

[47] Lefaucheur J, Drouot X, Nguyen J. Interventional neurophysiology for pain control: duration of pain relief following repetitive transcranial magnetic stimulation of the motor cortex. Neurophysiol Clin 2001;31:247-52.

[48] Rollnik J, Wüstefeld S, Däuper J, Karst M, Fink M, Kossev A, Dengler R. Repetitive transcranial magnetic stimulation for the treatment of chronic pain-A pilot study. Eur Neurol 2002;48:6-10.

[49] Lefaucheur J, Drouot X, Menard-Lefaucheur I, Zerah F, Bendib B, Cesaro P, et al. Neurogenic pain relief by repetitive transcranial magnetic cortical stimulation depends on the origin and the site of pain. J Neurol Neurosurg Psychiatry 2004;75:612-6.

[50] Khedr E, Kotb H, Kamel N, Ahmed M, Sadek R, Rothwell J. Long-lasting antalgic effects of daily sessions of repetitive transcranial magnetic stimulation in central and peripheral neuropathic pain. J Neurol Neurosurg Psychiatry 2005;76:833-8.

[51] Lefaucheur J, Hatem S, Nineb A, Menard-Lefaucheur I, Wendling S, Karavel Y, Nguyen J. Somatotopic organization of the analgesic effects of motor cortex rTMS in neuropathic pain. Neurology 2006;67:1998-2004.

[52] Hirayama A, Saitoh Y, Kishima H, Shimokawa T, Oshino S, Hirata M, et al. Reduction of intractable deafferentation pain by navigation-guided repetitive transcranial magnetic stimulation of the primary motor cortex. Pain 2006;122:22-7.

[53] André-Obadia N, Peyron R, Mertens P, Mauguière F, Laurent B, Garcia-Larrea L. Transcranial magnetic stimulation for pain control. Double-blind study of different frequencies against placebo, and correlation with motor cortex stimulation efficacy. Clin Neurophysiol 2006;117:1536-44.

[54] André-Obadia N, Mertens P, Gueguen A, Peyron R, Garcia-Larrea L. Pain relief by rTMS: Differential effect of current flow but no specific action on pain subtypes. Neurology 2008;71:833-40.

[55] Zaghi S, DaSilva AF, Acar M, Lopes M, Fregni F. One-year rTMS treatment for refractory trigeminal neuralgia. J Pain Symptom Manage 2009;38(4):1-5.

[56] Knotkova H. Transcranial direct current stimulation for the treatment of neuropathic pain. Oral presentation at Symposium: Brain stimulation in the treatment of chronic neuropathic pain: Deep brain stimulation, non-invasive stimulation or both? APS Meeting Tampa FL, 2009.

Chapter IX

Neuroplasticity in carpal tunnel syndrome

*Vitaly Napadow, PhD[*1,2], Yumi Maeda, PhD[1,2], Joseph Audette, MD[3,4] and Norman Kettner, DC[2]*

[1]Martinos Center for Biomedical Imaging, Department of Radiology, Massachusetts General Hospital, Charlestown, MA, US

[2]Department of Radiology, Logan College of Chiropractic, Chesterfield, MO, US

[3]Department of Pain Medicine, Harvard Vanguard Medical Associates, Atrius Health, Boston, MA, US

[4]Department of Physical Medicine and Rehabilitation, Spaulding Rehabilitation Hospital, Medford, MA, US

Abstract

Carpal tunnel syndrome (CTS) is the most common entrapment neuropathy. Compression of the peripheral median nerve within the carpal tunnel at the wrist leads to a range of structural and functional changes, which ultimately leads to neuroplastic change in the central nervous system (CNS). CTS is characterized by dysesthesias, or unpleasant atypical sensations, and persistent pain. This symptomatology

---

[*] Correspondence: Vitaly Napadow, PhD, Martinos Center for Biomedical Imaging, 149 Thirteenth St. #2301, Charlestown, MA 02129; E-mail: vitaly@nmr.mgh.harvard.edu

and peripheral nerve block change the quantity and quality of the somatosensory afference reaching the cortex, likely engendering central neuroplasticity. In fact, CTS provides an excellent opportunity to investigate cortical reorganization induced by clinically relevant aberrant afference in humans. Recent neuroimaging studies have applied techniques such as functional MRI (fMRI) and magnetoencephalography (MEG) to evaluate neuroplasticity in primary somatosensory cortex (SI) and elsewhere in the brain. This review will outline both peripheral pathophysiology characterizing chronic nerve compression, and the downstream central neuroplasticity that occurs with CTS and related nerve compression disorders. We will also detail therapeutic interventions that have demonstrated benefit for CTS. While surgery remains the definitive treatment for severe CTS, mild and moderate CTS may be treated with more conservative therapies, such as neuromodulation-based techniques, including TENS and electro-acupuncture. This review will also detail future directions for exploring neuroplasticity in CTS, as well as how better characterization of neuroplastic change in the CNS can inform the development of future therapeutic interventions.

Introduction

Carpal tunnel syndrome (CTS) is the most common entrapment neuropathy. Compression of the peripheral median nerve leads to a range of structural and functional changes, which ultimately leads to neuroplastic change in the central nervous system (CNS). Thus, while CTS is usually thought of as a peripheral nerve condition, central neuroplasticity has recently been described as well. This review will outline both the peripheral pathophysiology and the resultant central neuroplastic changes that occur with CTS and related nerve compression disorders.

CTS is only exceeded by low back pain as a cause of employee absenteeism (1). A recent cross-sectional study revealed a U.S. prevalence of 3.72% (2). In 1996 there was an estimated average treatment cost of $12,000 due to surgical intervention with total cost estimated at between 12-24 billion dollars per year (3).

Medical conditions associated with chronic CTS can include obesity, pregnancy, osteoarthritis, diabetes mellitus, amyloidosis, hypothyroidism, acromegaly, and use of corticosteroids and estrogens (4-8). Acute CTS is unusual and can result from a fracture of the distal radius (9). Occupationally, CTS is also associated with forceful repetitive activities of the hand and wrist (10). Factors that significantly increase the risk for CTS in the dominant hand of industrial workers include higher age, female gender, obesity, cigarette smoking, and use of vibration tools (6).

The exact criteria for the diagnosis of CTS, however, are not completely defined, and normal electrophysiological studies do not necessarily rule out CTS (11). Nevertheless, a consensus conference was organized that identified a combination of symptoms (numbness, tingling, burning and pain in combination with nocturnal symptoms) plus abnormal median nerve function based upon nerve conduction studies (NCS) as the 'gold standard' for the diagnosis of CTS (12). You et al. prospectively evaluated CTS patients (defined by NCS) and found significant correlations (P<0.001) for what they labeled as 'primary symptoms' (numbness, tingling, and nocturnal symptoms) and abnormal NCS (13). Other diagnostic approaches for CTS have included magnetic resonance imaging (MRI) (14) and ultrasound (US) (15, 16) evaluation of the median nerve and adjacent structures.

The key pathophysiologic variable in CTS is compression of the distal median nerve by an elevated pressure in the carpal tunnel usually secondary to flexor tenosynovitis (17). However, the chronic pathologic change involves fibrotic response to compression injury and CTS has been hypothesized to be more of an "–osis", rather than an inflammatory "–itis" (18). Injury to the median nerve induces a range of sensory symptoms primarily in the first through third digit and half of the fourth, spontaneous hand pain, nocturnal paresthesia, and hyperalgesia. In fact, paresthesias represent the most common symptom (19) and result from ectopic impulse activity generated by ischemic nerve damage (20, 21). Hand weakness, loss of fine coordination, and/or atrophy (in more severe cases) may also be present (22). Ultimately, there is a wide range of pathophysiological changes following peripheral nerve injury that include biochemical alterations, changes in gene expression, ion channel expression and synaptic function (23-25). The presence of persistent peripheral and central sensitization in spinal and supraspinal circuits is likely important in the development of chronic pain (26). Neuroplastic change or reorganization in cortical topography is either induced by increased neural activity (pain and paresthesia) or, in extremely severe cases, reduced activity from denervation.

Surgery is still considered the most definitive treatment with as high as 70-90% of patients reporting freedom from nocturnal pain after surgery (27). Nevertheless, surgery drives up costs and at least one follow up study suggested that patients who have undergone carpal tunnel release do no better than those who have been managed with conservative care (28). A recent review by O'Connor found that current evidence suggests short term benefit can be derived from a variety of conservative treatments, including oral steroids, splinting, ultrasound, yoga and carpal bone mobilization, but the durability of these treatments is not well known (29, 30). Recently, acupuncture has been reported to provide symptomatic relief (31, 32), and possibly improvement in nerve function (33).

In this review, we will focus on both the local pathophysiology and the concomitant central neuroplasticity found in CTS. We will address the following: 1) the peripheral pathophysiology that leads to neuroplastic change in the cortex, 2) central neuroplasticity including functional neuroimaging evidence, 3) neuroplastic change following neuromodulation and more conventional therapies, and 4) future directions in basic, clinical, and translational research. In order to broaden our scope somewhat, we will also refer to related disorders of nerve compression from both clinical and experimental animal models.

Peripheral pathophysiology underlying central neuroplasticity in CTS

Research into the pathophysiology of CTS has predominantly focused on peripheral nerve structure and function. Central neuroplasticity in the spinal cord and brain occurs in response to the peripheral nerve lesion in CTS. Thus, an appreciation of the peripheral pathophysiology in CTS and related nerve compression disorders is warranted.

The symptomatology and clinical findings of CTS are thought to result from chronic median nerve compression within the carpal tunnel. This compression is part of a vicious cycle of events that causes, via positive feedback, increased mechanical stress on the median nerve (Figure 1).

Increased pressure in the carpal tunnel compresses the median nerve, leads to ischemia and reperfusion injury from the release of free radicals, thus further damaging the nerve microvasculature (18). This damage then produces exudative edema and, chronically, results in fibrosis, which further increases the pressure within the carpal tunnel, cycling back again to produce more ischemia and so on. Ultimately, compression and the resultant cascade of pathologic changes produce positive symptomatology (e.g. paresthesias, pain) in the hand and median nerve innervated digits ($1^{st} - 4^{th}$).

In fact, CTS is associated with a broad symptomatology including paresthesias, pain, numbness, and weakness. Interestingly, paresthesias and nocturnal symptomatology (considered as "primary symptoms") may be more closely related to nerve function and median nerve conduction block than pain and weakness (considered as "secondary symptoms") (13).

In fact, electrophysiological testing in animal nerve compression models has found increased spiking along the nerve (34), which may be associated with paresthesia sensation in humans. Hence, it is possible that pain and paresthesias may be generated by different peripheral and/or central pathways in CTS.

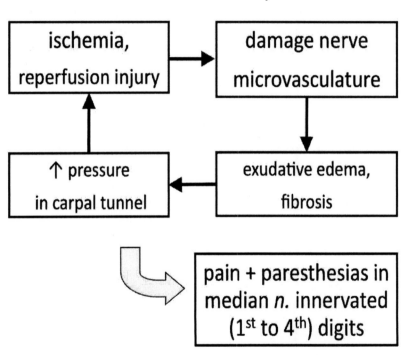

Figure 1. The vicious cycle underlying Carpal Tunnel Syndrome (CTS) results from pathophysiological and biochemical changes following an increase in pressure inside the carpal tunnel at the wrist. This increase in pressure compresses the median nerve, leading to ischemia and reperfusion injury, which damages the nerve microvasculature. This damage then produces exudative edema and fibrosis, which further increases the pressure inside the carpal tunnel, cycling back again to produce more ischemia etc. Ultimately, the compression and resultant pathological changes produce symptomatology (e.g. pain, paresthesias, numbness) in the hand and median nerve innervated digits.

CTS is significantly more prevalent in females than in males (35, 36). While this gender difference may be due to different geometry of the carpal tunnel, recent studies have also found increased expression of estrogen receptors (ER-α, ER-β) in the tenosynovium of postmenopousal females with CTS (37). More research is needed to understand the pathophysiology underlying the stark gender differences evident in CTS.

In addition to the characteristic symptomatology that occurs with CTS, nerve function itself is compromised. The most direct way to assess the CTS-associated conduction block is via electrophysiological testing. Many studies have now characterized the diminished velocities (latency prolongation) and amplitudes of an impulse traveling over the median nerve (13, 38-40). Both sensory and motor axons are affected, perhaps even in mild CTS (41). Interestingly, extra-median spread of nerve dysfunction has also been reported, specifically related to the ulnar nerve (42), which may explain the occasional extra-median spread of paresthesias and pain in CTS patients.

Given that a significant percentage of NCS for CTS produce false negative exams, imaging modalities have been used to increase diagnostic accuracy. Gross structural changes in the median nerve have been reported with imaging modalities such as ultrasound (15) and MRI (43). Ultrasonography has been employed for the diagnosis of CTS and showed significantly increased median nerve cross-sectional area (CSA) at the pisiform level, longitudinal compression signs and retinacular bowing (15). Of these parameters, the median nerve CSA at the pisiform level had a sensitivity of 82% and a specificity of 87.5%. In fact, the diagnostic accuracy of sonography is competitive with NCS (44). Studies have reported MRI sensitivity of 96%, and specificity of 33-38% for CTS (14). MR neurography, using fat-suppressed fluid-sensitive pulse sequences, has demonstrated proximal nerve swelling, increased flattening of the distal median nerve, and loss of MR signal along the nerve in the distal carpal tunnel (45). Diffusion tensor imaging (DTI), is an MRI method sensitive to molecular water diffusion along the nerve fiber. DTI provides quantitative in-vivo measures of axonal pathology (46). The number and length of tracked fibers, fractional anisotropy (FA) and apparent diffusion coefficient (ADC) of the median nerve in CTS was compared to 20 healthy controls and showed that mean FA value was 2 standard deviations below FA values in healthy controls, likely due to increased fibrosis which disrupts longitudinal (anisotropic) diffusion along the course of the median nerve (47).

Investigations of cellular and biochemical change at the lesion in both animals and humans have led to the hypothesis that CTS is a disease characterized more by chronic fibrosis, rather than chronic inflammation (18, 48). Histological evaluation of tenosynovial specimens from 41 patients who underwent carpel tunnel release surgery demonstrated edema and fibrous hypertrophy and fibroblast infiltration, but a lack of inflammatory cells (49). This result has now been corroborated by a different group (48), while increased edema (50) and vascular proliferation (51) have also been noted. Furthermore, immunohistological examination demonstrated increased production of IL-6 within endothelial cells (IL-6 plays a role in multiple non-inflammatory processes (52)) and prostaglandin E (PGE), but did not show increased IL-1 production. This same group also recently found evidence for tenosynovial connective tissue growth factor (CTGF) in a surgical sample from CTS patients (53), particularly in patients with co-morbid systemic lupus erythematosus (SLE) and rheumatoid arthritis (RA). Further research needs to elucidate just how strong of a role fibrosis actually plays in more common "idiopathic" CTS, without such rheumatological co-morbidities. Partially corroborative evidence has recently been provided by Frieboes et al. who used a rat sciatic nerve model (CCI) to demonstrate that while chronic nerve compression induces c-fos gene upregulation in the spinal dorsal horn, as well as Na_v 1.8 sodium channel expression in endoneurial Schwann cells, there was no evidence of increased TNF-α or IL-6 (54). Based on this evidence, the authors suggest that CTS is akin to non-inflammatory neuropathic pain rather than due to chronic inflammation. Regardless, the genetic and ion channel up-regulation suggested by these studies strongly implicate peripheral sensitization in CTS and related nerve compression disorders. Moreover, these same authors have also demonstrated an increase in the number of Schwann cells showing signs of apoptosis, axonal degeneration and axonal swelling in the CCI model (55). Furthermore, compressed nerves show decreased thickness of myelin, axon diameter and intermodal length (56). Thus the increased cross-sectional area of the median nerve apparent on ultrasound (15) and MRI (45) in CTS (mentioned above) is likely a function of intraneural edema and chronic fibrotic change within and around the peripheral median nerve.

Finally, several median nerve compression models relevant to CTS have been investigated in animals. Balloon catheter implantation in rabbit median nerve serves to increase pressure in the carpal tunnel. This compression can increase motor latency in a parametric pressure-dependent manner (57). A perhaps more clinically relevant rabbit model successfully increased pressure following hypertonic dextrose injection into the tenosynovium (subsynovial connective tissue) around the median nerve. This led to decreased motor conduction velocities and amplitudes, and produced proliferation of collagen within this subsynovial tissue (58). Thus, these models enter into the CTS vicious cycle at different points, but ultimately show that increased pressure and fibrosis produce nerve swelling, leading to sensory and motor conduction block over the median nerve, similar to that seen in the human syndrome.

Evidence of central neuroplasticity in CTS

Central neural plasticity is observed during development as well as learning (59). Environmental (exteroceptive and interoceptive) inputs shape the connectivity of the brain in both physiological and pathological states via known neuroplastic mechanisms (60). Do these mechanisms also play a role in CTS?

Several lines of evidence suggest that neuroplastic reorganization may contribute to the symptomatology and etiology of chronic CTS (61-64). For instance, Tinazzi et al. used somatosensory evoked potentials (SEPs) to demonstrate amplified neural response at multiple levels of the somatosensory processing system – spinal, brainstem, and cortex (64). However, many investigations of CTS neuroplasticity have focused more specifically on the primary somatosensory (SI) cortex (61-64).

The cortical representation of the hand and its digits in SI occupy a disproportionately large area of the somatotopic map, reflecting the density of sensory receptors peripherally located in the hand (65). The digits are represented in SI in sequential order, from digit 1 (D1) located ventrolaterally to digit 5 (D5) located more dorsomedially along the post-central gyrus. Many studies have found altered somatotopic organization of digits associated with increased, decreased, or aberrant somatosensory afference in both animals (66-68) and humans (69, 70). Cortical neuroplasticity specific to digit somatotopy has been investigated following experimentally decreased and aberrant sensory signaling. Substantial evidence supports the view that neuronal networks adjacent to a deafferented territory in SI may assume the function previously provided by deafferented neurons (71-73). For example, decreased sensory input induced by digit amputation or median nerve section in animal models results in the invasion of deafferented primary sensory cortical fields by the adjacent fields for intact digits (71, 72, 74). Moreover, electrophysiology studies demonstrate that surgically fusing adjacent digits blurs the affected digits' cortical representations in SI (66, 67). Such investigations of syndactyly, or the skin fold fusion of adjacent digits, suggest that neuroplasticity occurs due to afferent impulses from fused digits becoming more closely synchronized temporally compared with normally separated digits. Interestingly, similar results were obtained by training a monkey with temporally coherent multi-digit stimulation (68).

While the mechanisms underlying these neuroplastic responses are not entirely clear, the time scale for different forms of plasticity likely varies from minutes to years. The short term mechanism for wider cortical representations in physiological states has been attributed to a state of "disinhibition" (74). As the concentration of γ-aminobutyric acid (GABA) decreases in the cortex, existing "latent" subthreshold thalamocortical and cortico-cortical excitatory inputs are released from inhibitory control (75-77). Such short term neuroplastic changes may be reinforced over time with longer acting mechanisms via amplification of synaptic plasticity related to voltage gated, N-methyl-d-aspartate (NMDA) receptor mediated long term potentiation, or LTP (78, 79).

Thus, synaptic plasticity in CTS patients following aberrant somatosensory afference may be similar to "use-dependent plasticity" observed in many experimental models (80, 81). Temporally correlated synaptic activity increases the likelihood of long-lasting neural interactions or neuroplasticity (neurons that fire together, wire together) (82, 83).

CTS is characterized by dysesthesias, or unpleasant atypical sensations, and persistent pain. This symptomatology and the altered nerve conduction properties change the quantity and quality of the somatosensory afference reaching the cortex, likely engendering central neuroplasticity. In fact, CTS provides an excellent opportunity to investigate cortical reorganization induced by clinically relevant aberrant afference in humans.

Neuroimaging studies have used magnetoencephalography (MEG) and fMRI to evaluate SI neuroplasticity in CTS. Tecchio et al. used MEG to demonstrate amplified M30/M20 ratios following electrical stimulation of the median nerve and median nerve-innervated digits (63). Furthermore, the cortical representation of the affected hand (D1 to D5 separation distance) showed a more extended representation when paresthesias prevailed and contracted representation when pain was dominant. The authors hypothesized that the amplified cortical response was compensatory to reduced tactile information from the peripheral receptors subserving median nerve innervated digits. Napadow et al. used fMRI to map the SI response to electrical stimulation of both median and ulnar nerve innervated digits and found increased extent of activation for median nerve innervated D2 and D3 but not for ulnar nerve innervated D5 (62). Furthermore, SI somatotopy was also altered in CTS. The separation between cortical representations for D2 and D3 was closer in CTS patients compared to healthy adults, suggesting blurred cortical representations. Moreover, the D2/D3 separation distance was negatively correlated with nerve conduction latency — i.e., the worse the peripheral nerve dysfunction, the less separation between D2 and D3, thereby suggesting a stronger linkage between SI neuroplasticity and peripheral nerve (dys)function (Figure 2).

The authors hypothesized that blurred D2/D3 cortical representations may have been caused by the presence of paresthesias and explained by mechanisms of synaptic strengthening and cortical reorganization.

In CTS, paresthesias diffusely spread over D1 to D4, and thus are characterized by afference with greater temporal coherence across digits than is normally experienced. This temporal synchrony (which, as an aside, is also considered to be critical in formation of SI somatotopy during development (84)) strengthens synaptic connections, and may also lead to disinhibition of latent thalamo-cortical and cortico-cortical connections, which in turn leads to hyper-activated and blurred digit representations (Figure 3).

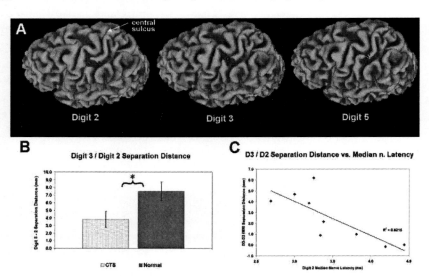

Figure 2. Neuroplasticity in CTS is found in primary somatosensory cortex (SI). (A) fMRI can be used to localize cortical digit representations in the post-central gyrus, or SI (center of mass is superimposed over hand area SI activations from a representative subject). (B) The digit 3 / digit 2 (D3/D2) separation distance is closer for CTS patients compared to controls. (C) D3 / D2 separation distance is negatively correlated with median nerve latency – the worse the peripheral nerve dysfunction, the closer the D3 / D2 separation distance. Adapted from (62).

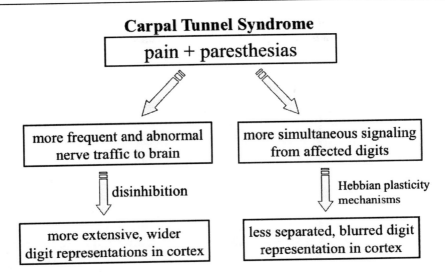

Figure 3. In CTS, pain and paresthesias diffusely spread over D1 to D4, and thus are characterized by afference with greater temporal coherence across digits than is normally experienced. This temporal synchrony strengthens synaptic connections via Hebbian plasticity and may lead to disinhibition of latent thalamo-cortical and cortico-cortical connections. These neuroplastic changes manifest in hyper-activated and blurred SI digit representations in neuroimaging investigations of CTS patients.

Ultimately, these neuroimaging results corroborate the hypothesis that CTS includes a central neuroplastic manifestation of a peripheral lesion.

Interestingly, recent studies have suggested that cortical disinhibition in CTS may be more widespread than previously thought, and not just confined to SI representations of median nerve innervated digits, or even SI. For example, pressure pain threshold (PPT) testing is lowered bilaterally in the hand and proximal to the wrist in unilateral CTS (85, 86). Similarly, heat/cold pain threshold is also lowered bilaterally in the hand/wrist in the patients with unilateral CTS (87). Moreover, recent reports suggest that pathological change following median nerve compression is not limited to median nerve innervated territory, but may become extraterritorial involving territory innervated by both ulnar and radial nerves, which are adjacent in higher cortical and subcortical somatosensory areas (88, 89).

Additionally, the presence of chronic pain in CTS raises intriguing questions regarding additional interactions with neuroplastic mechanisms noted for other chronic pain conditions. Impaired cognition has been described in chronic pain disorders (90). Furthermore, cortical representation of an affected body part (back representation) in patients with chronic low back pain was reported shifting medially towards the hip (91). In MEG studies of CRPS 1, the representations of D1 and D5 were closer to one another on the affected hand (92, 93), with cortical reorganization (expressed as the lip to D1/D5 midpoint relative distance) correlating with extent of hyperalgesia (93).

Neuroplasticity outside of SI has also been suggested by prior studies. Napadow et al. noted increased activation in precentral gyrus and dorsolateral prefrontal cortex following somatosensory stimulation of median nerve affected digits – suggesting upregulated interactions between somatosensory and (a) primary motor and (b) higher cognitive brain regions (62). Motor planning areas may also be affected. Though motor loss in CTS is a late clinical finding, hand weakness and clumsiness have been reported in 56% and 48% of CTS respectively (94). Slowing of motor planning/execution and lack of fine motor control have been assessed by a "psychomotor" performance task (PMP), which used a pinch grip test with visual feedback to evaluate the initiation and fine control of muscles innervated by the median nerve motor branch. CTS patients showed decreased pinch strength (28%), slower controlled pinch performance (24%) and greater pinch limit overshoot (76%) (95). Thus, the SI neuroplasticity observed in CTS may also influence subsequent processing in other brain regions (e.g., cognitive, autonomic, affective).

Treatment of CTS and accompanied neuroplasticity

Several treatment options exist for CTS (31). Most of these therapies are focused on changing the biomechanics and hemodynamics local to the lesion at the wrist (96, 97). However, as discussed above, central neuroplasticity may also be an important factor in CTS symptomatology and conservative neuromodulatory treatment approaches may play a role in the eventual abatement of symptoms such as pain and paresthesias. While research on this topic has been scant, a brief review is justified and will be included following a discourse on more conventional therapeutic approaches.

Surgery is considered a definitive treatment for CTS, with as high as 70–90% of subjects reporting freedom from nocturnal pain after both endoscopic and open carpal tunnel release surgery (27). A long term follow up study has shown that patients maintain symptom/ performance improvements with high satisfaction (94%) 5 years following surgery (98). Surgery has also been shown to affect complex task performance attributed to higher brain functioning, likely as a result of neuroplasticity in the CNS. These effects may have resulted from enhanced sensory feedback following improvement in peripheral nerve function. For example, gap detection testing improved 43% and pinch/release rate in the PMP test improved by 20% following carpal tunnel release (99). Control CTS patients who did not undergo surgery showed no improvement in gap detection and only 7% improvement in pinch/release rate (likely due to test-retest motor learning). Similarly, Hsu et al. recently found that surgery improved not just two-point discrimination and Semmes-Weinstein pressure thresholds (likely due to neuroplasticity in SI), but also more complex tests of dexterity, such as a pinch holding test (100), which involves neuroplasticity in brain regions subserving sensorimotor coupling and fine motor control.

While surgery is the most definitive treatment for severe CTS, not all patients respond favorably. Post-surgical allodynia rates have been reported to be as high as 6-41% 1 month to 1 year after open surgical decompression (101). Positive Tinel's sign (5%), scar tenderness (7%) and pillar pain (12%) have also been reported following surgery (102). Surgical outcome may hinge on multiple factors, and worse outcomes have been related to pre-surgery upper extremity functional limitation, poor mental health status, alcohol use, and the involvement of an attorney (10). Similarly, in patients with upper limb peripheral nerve transection, chronic neuropathic pain following surgical repair of median and/or ulnar nerve transection was more prevalent in patients with increased pain catastrophizing, but also poor pre-surgical performance on sensorimotor integration tasks (103). These results suggest that neuroplasticity in the brain is not only a central response to peripheral nerve lesions, but can also influence response to therapy. However, surgery drives up costs and at least one follow up study has suggested that patients who have undergone carpal tunnel release do no better than those who have been managed with conservative care. Specifically, when splinting (see below) was compared to surgical carpal tunnel release, follow up demonstrated no significant difference in symptomatology and function (e.g. 2-point discrimination, grip strength) between the two (28).

A broad range of conservative treatments have been used to mollify the symptoms of CTS (29). In addition, a review by O'Connor et al. (30) found that the evidence to date suggested that short term benefit can be derived from oral steroids, splinting, ultrasound, yoga, and carpal bone mobilization, though the durability of these treatments was not known. One of the most common approaches is splinting of the wrist, which helps to keep the wrist in a neutral position, lowering the pressure in the carpal tunnel (104) and producing symptom relief (105). Use of a nocturnal wrist brace has produced significant improvement in symptoms and function compared to no treatment following 4 weeks of use (106), as well as 3 months use (30, 107, 108). Although no improvements of electrophysiological measurements has been reported in short term use (106), a long term follow up study showed splinting did provide symptomatic relief and improved sensory and motor conduction velocity when the patient wore splints every night (109). However, splinting may not produce added improvement following surgery. For example, 3 months follow up demonstrated no significant difference in symptomatology and function (e.g. 2-point discrimination, grip strength) between post-operative splinting for 2 days versus the use of bandages (28). Both splinting and surgery suppress the pressure inside the carpal tunnel, though the suppression is likely much greater in surgery compared to splinting. Therefore, treatment should be determined according to the severity of nerve compression, and splinting may be preferable in mild and moderate CTS.

Another conservative approach has been local corticosteroid injection, which improved symptoms in more than 70% of patients, with short term improvement in median nerve conduction (110, 111). However, symptoms generally recur within 1 year (109). An unblinded randomized clinical trial demonstrated that corticosteroid injection compared to NSAIDs plus splinting produced similar improvements in symptom severity and nerve conduction latency at 8 weeks (112). Corticosteroid injection or oral steroids have also been used to suppress pain, conceivably through anti-inflammatory mechanisms, affecting nociception at the spinal and supraspinal level (113).

Acupuncture has also been applied as a conservative treatment for CTS. A recent meta-analysis, while somewhat premature given the number of published trials, found that the evidence supporting acupuncture as a symptomatic therapy for CTS is encouraging (114). Different forms of acupuncture (e.g. manual vs. electro-acupuncture) likely provide significantly different degrees of neuromodulatory input to the peripheral and central nervous system. Notwithstanding, acupuncture has been shown to affect both symptomatology and more objective outcome measures such as NCS. Naeser et al. found a significant reduction in pain and median nerve sensory latency after a mixed laser acupuncture/micro transcutaneous electrical nerve stimulation (Micro-TENS) treatment protocol compared to sham stimulation in a crossover design trial (115). In an un-controlled study, Chen et al. also reported symptom relief using both manual and electrical acupuncture (116).

More recently, Yang et al. demonstrated in a randomized controlled trial that a 4 week trial of manual acupuncture local to the lesion demonstrated greater improvement in symptomatology (e.g. nocturnal awakening) and nerve conduction (e.g. distal motor latency) compared to oral steroid use (32). Other symptom scores and nerve conduction tests were equally improved after both active therapies. As there were minimal adverse events during acupuncture, the authors concluded that acupuncture is a viable alternative for those who have intolerance or contraindication for oral steroid or for those not opting for surgery.

Although the mechanisms by which acupuncture affects CTS are not well understood, a recent study suggests that modulation of neuroplasticity may play a role. Napadow et al. used fMRI, an imaging modality that can non-invasively map digit somatotopy (117-119), to assess cortical reorganization in CTS patients post-acupuncture (33). FMRI was also used to correlate these changes with the degree of clinical improvement. Therapy included both low frequency (2Hz) electro-acupuncture local to the lesion, and manual acupuncture at both proximal and distal forearm acupoints. The authors found that the previously demonstrated (62) cortical hyperactivation to non-noxious stimuli in CTS patients was diminished for D3 after a 5 week course of acupuncture treatment (Figure 4).

Furthermore, the separation between D3 and D2 cortical representations in SI, which was contracted in CTS patients (62), increased after acupuncture therapy (Figure 4). Moreover, the increase in D3/D2 separation correlated with improvement in both median nerve sensory conduction latency and reported paresthesias. Recently, TENS treatment at similar forearm locations was also found to diminish sensorimotor activation, in this case acutely (120). In summary, these data suggest a beneficial cortical plasticity associated with improved CTS symptomatology following acupuncture, and potentially TENS, therapy.

Just how acupuncture induces neuroplasticity is unknown. For instance, cortical neuroplastic change may occur as a consequence of improvement in peripheral nerve function. Acupuncture is known to up-regulate local blood flow (121), likely through the stimulated release of vasodilatory peptides such as calcitonin gene-regulated peptide (CGRP) (122-124). Peripherally addressing the ischemic insult could then modify the maladaptive neuroplasticity seen in CTS. However, acupuncture may also drive neuroplasticity in the sensorimotor cortex directly via modulation in subcortical-cortical (e.g. limbic, see (125-128)) and/or cortico-cortical circuits to relieve symptomatology maintained by brain circuitry. Acupuncture, and other sensory conditioning stimuli, may modulate the CNS directly through classic spinal-thalamic (129) or indirectly through spino-limbic-cortical pathways (130, 131). In fact, SI receives robust projections from limbic regions including the amygdala (132, 133), and amygdaloid projections to primary sensory cortices are more widespread than cortico-amygdaloid projections (134). Moreover, cortical sensory regions demonstrate enhanced response during exposure to emotionally valenced sensory stimuli (135, 136). In turn, acupuncture has been shown to down-regulate amygdala activity in human fMRI studies (125-128, 137) and in a study using chronically implanted recording electrodes in monkeys (138). Furthermore, acupuncture induces greater amygdala deactivation and hypothalamic activation in CTS patients compared to healthy controls (139).

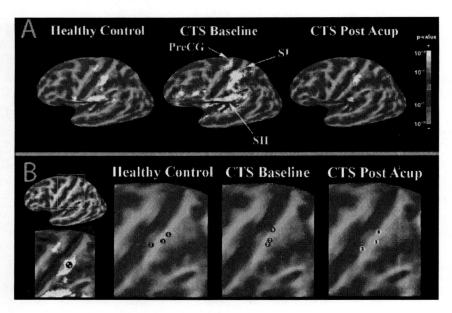

Figure 4. (A) Functional MRI (fMRI) has recently demonstrated that CTS leads to hyperactivation of primary somatosensory cortex (SI) and other brain structures in response to electrical stimulation for digit 3 (D3), a median nerve innervated digit. Following treatment with acupuncture, hyperactivation was found to decrease. (B) Multi-digit stimulation found that CTS is also characterized by aberrant somatotopy in SI, where median nerve innervated digits 2 (D2) and D3 have cortical receptive fields with center-of-mass closer to one another, compared to healthy adults. Again, treatment with acupuncture was found to increase this D3 / D2 separation distance. Adapted from (33, 62).

Thus, acupuncture, as a combination of somatosensory conditioning stimuli with a uniquely salient, affective context, may also modulate neuroplasticity in SI via limbic-cortical projections. However, the most likely scenario is that acupuncture modulates cortical neuroplasticity both directly, through central processing of acupuncture stimuli, and indirectly, through sensory conditioning of the peripheral median nerve.

Future directions

While several viable options exist for both conservative and surgical treatment of CTS and related nerve compression disorders, CNS neuroplasticity may present another target for neuromodulatory therapies. Neuroplastic modulation using patterned sensorimotor stimulation is a promising technique for neurological rehabilitation. These approaches are dependent in part on the evolution of our understanding of cortical sensorimotor synaptic plasticity. The management of neurological and behavioral disorders, particularly disorders which involve sensory learning, will incorporate an understanding and therapeutic manipulation of somatotopy and sensorimotor synaptic plasticity.

In addition, from the standpoint of basic science, clarification of the spatial and temporal mechanisms underlying neural encoding at the cortical level would enhance our understanding of the dynamics of somatotopy and its reorganization. Recognition of the specific role and mechanisms of use (disuse)-dependent plasticity in the CNS would provide new insights into physiological and pathological states. New models elucidating the nature of spatiotemporal encoding in neuroplasticity could contribute to our understanding of cognitive systems such as memory and learning.

Synchronization of oscillatory neural activity underlies the capacity for communication across local and distributed neural networks. This is an important mechanism for the functions of cognition, memory and perception. One of the likely candidate mechanisms for the synchronization or de-synchronization of oscillatory neural activity may be spike timing dependent synaptic plasticity (STDP) (140, 141). This form of plasticity involves the capacity of neurons to modulate the strength of their synaptic connections (i.e. neuroplasticity) via relative timing of pre- and postsynaptic action potentials. Pathological synchronization of neural activity has been reported in several neurological disease states including pain, epilepsy and Parkinson's disease (142, 143). It may be that pathologically synchronized brain states develop an autonomous and isolated level of function, divorced from afferent input. Desynchronizing abnormal brain activity using high frequency deep brain stimulation has been used to reset and re-establish physiological synaptic activity (144). This principle employs weak sensory inputs that modify and restore the functional capacity of neuronal circuits, which, at least in the case of Parkinson's disease, have lost their segregated neural activity and have undergone abnormal synchronization (145).

The central neuroplasticity underlying chronic neuropathic pain and entrapment neuropathies such as CTS may also evidence pathological synchronization and, thus, similar de-synchronizing stimulation techniques applied in the periphery may modulate functionally abnormal brain oscillatory networks. More specifically, feedback approaches could be devised wherein oscillatory activity is measured in real-time by electroencephalography (EEG), and peripheral stimulation is applied (via TENS or acupuncture procedures) appropriately gated to the measured oscillatory activity in order to interrupt any pathological synchronization. Such an approach could be studied in the future as a way to optimize these therapies incorporating knowledge of brain neuroplasticity in CTS and related disorders.

The therapeutic manipulation of cortical neuroplastic reorganization may hold promise for the treatment of neuropathic pain and disease, including CTS, but also diabetes mellitus. The patient with diabetic neuropathy carries a significant burden of morbidity due to elevated risk for delayed recognition of trauma and infections, as the foot or hand is typically insensate. The use of a cutaneous anesthetic blockade in the lower leg has been shown to improve more distal sensation in healthy adults (146). Recently, in a randomized, double blind study, anesthetic cream was applied to the leg of diabetics (type I or II) for 1.5 hours. A significant improvement was seen in the touch threshold of plantar metatarsal sites along with a decreased vibration threshold (147). This therapeutic manipulation of cortical somatotopy was apparently created by the induction of a "cortical silent zone" following deafferentation of the leg by the topical anesthetic. This cortical silent zone prompted the expansion of adjacent (somatotopic) receptive fields in SI and an adaptive reorganization resulting in improved neuropathic sensory status (147). This application of therapeutic cortical reorganization may prove useful in other forms of neuropathic disease including neuropathic pain and CTS. Additional scientific investigation is clearly warranted.

The investigation of cortical neuroplastic reorganization in disuse has received less study than use-dependent plasticity. This is enigmatic as many pathological disorders and treatments are characterized by, or require, prolonged immobilization of a body part. Many studies evaluating use-dependent plasticity report enlargement of cortical somatotopic representations. This was seen with median nerve involved digits in CTS patients likely arising from prolonged paresthesia and or pain (62). In a recent study, the effects of a few weeks of hand and arm immobilization by a cast were studied using fMRI with comparison made to healthy controls (148). The finger somatotopy of the contralateral SI displayed reduced activation that correlated with hand-use frequency and the subject's impaired tactile acuity correlated with deactivation. These cortical and perceptual changes recovered after cast removal. There was, interestingly, a contralateral (non-casted) cortical compensation consisting of increased perceptual performance (tactile acuity) that persisted beyond the period of cast removal. This response on the non-casted side may have been related to use-dependent plasticity in compensation to increased demand.

The targeted therapeutic modulation of cortical somatotopic reorganization offers promise for a diverse range of disorders beyond peripheral neuropathy. This could include chronic pain disorders, neurodegenerative disease and possibly cognitive disorders that arise from altered perceptual function, such as anorexia and obesity. It is likely that the evolution of this field will continue to be fueled by basic science advances in the understanding neuroplasticity mechanisms along with the development of new structural and functional imaging techniques. It is clear that application of neuroplasticity-based therapies to treat neurological disease has been relatively limited and will be greatly surpassed in the near future.

Acknowledgment

We would like to thank the National Center for Complementary and Alternative Medicine, NIH for funding support: K01-AT002166, R01-AT004714 (Napadow), P01-AT002048 (Rosen). We also acknowledge the NCRR (P41-RR14075, GCRC M01-RR01066) and the Mental Illness and Neuroscience Discovery (MIND) Institute.

References

[1] Trumble TE, Gilbert M, McCallister WV. Endoscopic versus open surgical treatment of carpal tunnel syndrome. Neurosurg Clin North Am 2001;12(2):255-66.

[2] Papanicolaou GD, McCabe SJ, Firrell J. The prevalence and characteristics of nerve compression symptoms in the general population. J Hand Surg [Am] 2001;26(3):460-6.

[3] Clairmont A. Economic aspects of carpal tunnel syndrome. In: Kraft GH, Johnson EW, editors. Phys Med Rehabil Clin North Am 1997:571-6.

[4] Palumbo CF, Szabo RM, Olmsted SL. The effects of hypothyroidism and thyroid replacement on the development of carpal tunnel syndrome. J Hand Surg Am 2000;25(4):734-9.

[5] Solomon DH, Katz JN, Bohn R, Mogun H, Avorn J. Nonoccupational risk factors for carpal tunnel syndrome. J Gen Intern Med 1999;14(5):310-4.

[6] Nathan PA, Meadows KD, Istvan JA. Predictors of carpal tunnel syndrome: an 11-year study of industrial workers. J Hand Surg [Am] 2002;27(4):644-51.

[7] Nathan PA, Istvan JA, Meadows KD. A longitudinal study of predictors of research-defined carpal tunnel syndrome in industrial workers: findings at 17 years. J Hand Surg Br 2005;30(6):593-8.

[8] Ferry S, Hannaford P, Warskyj M, Lewis M, Croft P. Carpal tunnel syndrome: a nested case-control study of risk factors in women. Am J Epidemiol 2000;151(6):566-74.

[9] Geoghegan JM, Clark DI, Bainbridge LC, Smith C, Hubbard R. Risk factors in carpal tunnel syndrome. J Hand Surg Br 2004;29(4):315-20.

[10] Katz JN, Losina E, Amick BC, 3rd, Fossel AH, Bessette L, Keller RB. Predictors of outcomes of carpal tunnel release. Arthritis Rheum 2001;44(5):1184-93.

[11] Jablecki CK, Andary MT, So YT, Wilkins DE, Williams FH. Literature review of the usefulness of nerve conduction studies and electromyography for the evaluation of patients with carpal tunnel syndrome. AAEM Quality Assurance Committee. Muscle Nerve 1993;16(12):1392-414.

[12] Rempel D, Evanoff B, Amadio PC, de Krom M, Franklin G, Franzblau A, et al. Consensus criteria for the classification of carpal tunnel syndrome in epidemiologic studies. Am J Public Health 1998;88(10):1447-51.

[13] You H, Simmons Z, Freivalds A, Kothari MJ, Naidu SH. Relationships between clinical symptom severity scales and nerve conduction measures in carpal tunnel syndrome. Muscle Nerve 1999;22(4):497-501.

[14] Jarvik JG, Yuen E, Haynor DR, Bradley CM, Fulton-Kehoe D, Smith-Weller T, et al. MR nerve imaging in a prospective cohort of patients with suspected carpal tunnel syndrome. Neurology 2002;58(11):1597-602.

[15] Wang LY, Leong CP, Huang YC, Hung JW, Cheung SM, Pong YP. Best diagnostic criterion in high-resolution ultrasonography for carpal tunnel syndrome. Chang Gung Med J 2008;31(5):469-76.

[16] Chen YI, Wang FN, Nelson AJ, Xu H, Kim Y, Rosen BR, et al. Electrical stimulation modulates the amphetamine-induced hemodynamic changes: an fMRI study to compare the effect of stimulating locations and frequencies on rats. Neurosci Lett 2008;444(2):117-21.

[17] Sud V, Tucci MA, Freeland AE, Smith WT, Grinspun K. Absorptive properties of synovium harvested from the carpal tunnel. Microsurgery 2002;22(7):316-9.

[18] Sud V, Freeland AE. Biochemistry of carpal tunnel syndrome. Microsurgery 2005;25(1):44-6.

[19] Nora DB, Becker J, Ehlers JA, Gomes I. What symptoms are truly caused by median nerve compression in carpal tunnel syndrome? Clin Neurophysiol 2005;116(2):275-83.

[20] Mogyoros I, Bostock H, Burke D. Mechanisms of paresthesias arising from healthy axons. Muscle Nerve 2000;23(3):310-20.

[21] Ochoa JL, Torebjork HE. Paraesthesiae from ectopic impulse generation in human sensory nerves. Brain 1980;103(4):835-53.

[22] Stevens JC. AAEM minimonograph #26: the electrodiagnosis of carpal tunnel syndrome. American Association of Electrodiagnostic Medicine. Muscle Nerve 1997;20(12):1477-86.

[23] Zhang L, Xiao C, Wang JK, Zhang LC, Zeng YM. Activation of extracellular signal-regulated protein kinases 5 in the spinal cord contributes to the neuropathic pain behaviors induced by CCI in rats. Neurol Res 2009;31(10):1037-43.

[24] Buhrich N, Doutney C, Daniels P, Cohen A, Virgona A. Psychosocial profile of residents at a large hostel for homeless men. Med J Aust 1991;154(8):566.

[25] Staaf S, Oerther S, Lucas G, Mattsson JP, Ernfors P. Differential regulation of TRP channels in a rat model of neuropathic pain. Pain 2009;144(1-2):187-99.

[26] Latremoliere A, Woolf CJ. Central sensitization: a generator of pain hypersensitivity by central neural plasticity. J Pain 2009;10(9):895-926.

[27] Katz JN, Keller RB, Simmons BP, Rogers WD, Bessette L, Fossel AH, et al. Maine Carpal Tunnel Study: outcomes of operative and nonoperative therapy for carpal tunnel syndrome in a community-based cohort. J Hand Surg [Am] 1998;23(4):697-710.

[28] Huemer GM, Koller M, Pachinger T, Dunst KM, Schwarz B, Hintringer T. Postoperative splinting after open carpal tunnel release does not improve functional and neurological outcome. Muscle Nerve 2007;36(4):528-31.

[29] Wilson JK, Sevier TL. A review of treatment for carpal tunnel syndrome. Disabil Rehabil 2003;25(3):113-9.

[30] O'Connor D, Marshall S, Massy-Westropp N. Non-surgical treatment (other than steroid injection) for carpal tunnel syndrome. Cochrane Database Syst Rev 2003(1):CD003219.

[31] Carlson H, Colbert A, Frydl J, Arnall E, Elliot M, Carlson N. Current options for nonsurgical management of carpal tunnel syndrome. Int J Clin Rheumtol 2010;5(1):129-42.

[32] Yang CP, Hsieh CL, Wang NH, Li TC, Hwang KL, Yu SC, et al. Acupuncture in patients with carpal tunnel syndrome: A randomized controlled trial. Clin J Pain 2009;25(4):327-33.

[33] Napadow V, Liu J, Li M, Kettner N, Ryan A, Kwong KK, et al. Somatosensory cortical plasticity in carpal tunnel syndrome treated by acupuncture. Hum Brain Mapp 2007;28(3):159-71.

[34] Nakamura S, Atsuta Y. Electrophysiological study on primary afferent properties of a chronic constriction nerve injury model in spinal rats. J Orthop Sci 2004;9(4):386-91.

[35] de Krom MC, Knipschild PG, Kester AD, Thijs CT, Boekkooi PF, Spaans F. Carpal tunnel syndrome: prevalence in the general population. J Clin Epidemiol 1992;45(4):373-6.

[36] Bongers FJ, Schellevis FG, van den Bosch WJ, van der Zee J. Carpal tunnel syndrome in general practice (1987 and 2001): incidence and the role of occupational and non-occupational factors. Br J Gen Pract 2007;57(534):36-9.

[37] Kim JK, Hann HJ, Kim MJ, Kim JS. The expression of estrogen receptors in the tenosynovium of postmenopausal women with idiopathic carpal tunnel syndrome. J Orthop Res 2010;28(11):1469-74.

[38] Chang MH, Lee YC, Hsieh PF. The real role of forearm mixed nerve conduction velocity in the assessment of proximal forearm conduction slowing in carpal tunnel syndrome. J Clin Neurophysiol 2008;25(6):373-7.

[39] Chang MH, Lee YC, Hsieh PF. The role of forearm mixed nerve conduction study in the evaluation of proximal conduction slowing in carpal tunnel syndrome. Clin Neurophysiol 2008;119(12):2800-3.

[40] Chang MH, Liu LH, Lee YC, Hsieh PF. Alteration of proximal conduction velocity at distal nerve injury in carpal tunnel syndrome: demyelinating versus axonal change. J Clin Neurophysiol 2008;25(3):161-6.

[41] Ginanneschi F, Mondelli M, Dominici F, Rossi A. Changes in motor axon recruitment in the median nerve in mild carpal tunnel syndrome. Clin Neurophysiol 2006;117(11):2467-72.

[42] Ginanneschi F, Milani P, Mondelli M, Dominici F, Biasella A, Rossi A. Ulnar sensory nerve impairment at the wrist in carpal tunnel syndrome. Muscle Nerve 2008;37(2):183-9.

[43] Andreisek G, Crook DW, Burg D, Marincek B, Weishaupt D. Peripheral neuropathies of the median, radial, and ulnar nerves: MR imaging features. Radiographics 2006;26(5):1267-87.

[44] Visser LH, Smidt MH, Lee ML. High-resolution sonography versus EMG in the diagnosis of carpal tunnel syndrome. J Neurol Neurosurg Psychiatry 2008;79(1):63-7.

[45] Cudlip SA, Howe FA, Clifton A, Schwartz MS, Bell BA. Magnetic resonance neurography studies of the median nerve before and after carpal tunnel decompression. J Neurosurg 2002;96(6):1046-51.

[46] Kabakci NT, Kovanlikaya A, Kovanlikaya I. Tractography of the median nerve. Semin Musculoskelet Radiol 2009;13(1):18-23.

[47] Kabakci N, Gurses B, Firat Z, Bayram A, Ulug AM, Kovanlikaya A, et al. Diffusion tensor imaging and tractography of median nerve: normative diffusion values. AJR Am J Roentgenol 2007;189(4):923-7.

[48] Donato G, Galasso O, Valentino P, Conforti F, Zuccala V, Russo E, et al. Pathological findings in subsynovial connective tissue in idiopathic carpal tunnel syndrome. Clin Neuropathol 2009;28(2):129-35.

[49] Freeland AE, Tucci MA, Barbieri RA, Angel MF, Nick TG. Biochemical evaluation of serum and flexor tenosynovium in carpal tunnel syndrome. Microsurgery 2002;22(8):378-85.

[50] Fuchs PC, Nathan PA, Myers LD. Synovial histology in carpal tunnel syndrome. J Hand Surg Am 1991;16(4):753-8.

[51] Kim JK, Koh YD, Kim JS, Hann HJ, Kim MJ. Oxidative stress in subsynovial connective tissue of idiopathic carpal tunnel syndrome. J Orthop Res 2010;28(11):1463-8.

[52] Gauldie J, Richards C, Baumann H. IL6 and the acute phase reaction. Res Immunol 1992;143(7):755-9.

[53] Pierce CW, Tucci MA, Lindley S, Freeland A, Benghuzzi HA. Connective tissue growth factor (ctgf) expression in the tenosynovium of patients with carpal tunnel syndrome - biomed 2009. Biomed Sci Instrum 2009;45:30-5.

[54] Frieboes LR, Palispis WA, Gupta R. Nerve compression activates selective nociceptive pathways and upregulates peripheral sodium channel expression in Schwann cells. J Orthop Res 2010;28(6):753-61.

[55] Gupta R, Steward O. Chronic nerve compression induces concurrent apoptosis and proliferation of Schwann cells. J Comp Neurol 2003;461(2):174-86.

[56] Gupta R, Rowshan K, Chao T, Mozaffar T, Steward O. Chronic nerve compression induces local demyelination and remyelination in a rat model of carpal tunnel syndrome. Exp Neurol 2004;187(2):500-8.

[57] Diao E, Shao F, Liebenberg E, Rempel D, Lotz JC. Carpal tunnel pressure alters median nerve function in a dose-dependent manner: a rabbit model for carpal tunnel syndrome. J Orthop Res 2005;23(1):218-23.

[58] Yoshii Y, Zhao C, Schmelzer JD, Low PA, An KN, Amadio PC. The effects of hypertonic dextrose injection on connective tissue and nerve conduction through the rabbit carpal tunnel. Arch Phys Med Rehabil 2009;90(2):333-9.

[59] Galvan A. Neural plasticity of development and learning. Hum Brain Mapp 2010;31(6):879-90.

[60] Cohen S, Greenberg ME. Communication between the synapse and the nucleus in neuronal development, plasticity, and disease. Annu Rev Cell Dev Biol 2008;24:183-209.

[61] Druschky K, Kaltenhauser M, Hummel C, Druschky A, Huk WJ, Stefan H, et al. Alteration of the somatosensory cortical map in peripheral mononeuropathy due to carpal tunnel syndrome. Neuroreport 2000;11(17):3925-30.

[62] Napadow V, Kettner N, Ryan A, Kwong KK, Audette J, Hui KK. Somatosensory cortical plasticity in carpal tunnel syndrome--a cross-sectional fMRI evaluation. Neuroimage 2006;31(2):520-30.

[63] Tecchio F, Padua L, Aprile I, Rossini PM. Carpal tunnel syndrome modifies sensory hand cortical somatotopy: a MEG study. Hum Brain Mapp 2002;17(1):28-36.

[64] Tinazzi M, Zanette G, Volpato D, Testoni R, Bonato C, Manganotti P, et al. Neurophysiological evidence of neuroplasticity at multiple levels of the somatosensory system in patients with carpal tunnel syndrome. Brain 1998;121(Pt 9):1785-94.

[65] Penfield W, Boldrey E. Somatic motor and sensory representationin the cerebral cortex of man as studied by electrical stimulation. Brain 1937;60:389-443.

[66] Allard T, Clark SA, Jenkins WM, Merzenich MM. Reorganization of somatosensory area 3b representations in adult owl monkeys after digital syndactyly. J Neurophysiol 1991;66(3):1048-58.

[67] Clark SA, Allard T, Jenkins WM, Merzenich MM. Receptive fields in the body-surface map in adult cortex defined by temporally correlated inputs. Nature 1988;332(6163):444-5.

[68] Wang X, Merzenich MM, Sameshima K, Jenkins WM. Remodelling of hand representation in adult cortex determined by timing of tactile stimulation. Nature 1995;378(6552):71-5.

[69] Godde B, Spengler F, Dinse HR. Associative pairing of tactile stimulation induces somatosensory cortical reorganization in rats and humans. Neuroreport 1996;8(1):281-5.

[70] Pilz K, Veit R, Braun C, Godde B. Effects of co-activation on cortical organization and discrimination performance. Neuroreport 2004;15(17):2669-72.

[71] Merzenich MM, Nelson RJ, Stryker MP, Cynader MS, Schoppmann A, Zook JM. Somatosensory cortical map changes following digit amputation in adult monkeys. J Comp Neurol 1984;224(4):591-605.

[72] Merzenich MM, Kaas JH, Wall J, Nelson RJ, Sur M, Felleman D. Topographic reorganization of somatosensory cortical areas 3b and 1 in adult monkeys following restricted deafferentation. Neuroscience 1983;8(1):33-55.

[73] Kew JJ, Halligan PW, Marshall JC, Passingham RE, Rothwell JC, Ridding MC, et al. Abnormal access of axial vibrotactile input to deafferented somatosensory cortex in human upper limb amputees. J Neurophysiol 1997;77(5):2753-64.

[74] Calford MB, Tweedale R. Immediate and chronic changes in responses of somatosensory cortex in adult flying-fox after digit amputation. Nature 1988;332(6163):446-8.

[75] Levy LM, Ziemann U, Chen R, Cohen LG. Rapid modulation of GABA in sensorimotor cortex induced by acute deafferentation. Ann Neurol 2002;52(6):755-61.

[76] Jones EG. GABAergic neurons and their role in cortical plasticity in primates. Cereb Cortex 1993;3(5):361-72.

[77] Dykes RW. Mechanisms controlling neuronal plasticity in somatosensory cortex. Can J Physiol Pharmacol 1997;75(5):535-45.

[78] Brown TH, Chapman PF, Kairiss EW, Keenan CL. Long-term synaptic potentiation. Science 1988;242(4879):724-8.

[79] Buonomano DV, Merzenich MM. Cortical plasticity: from synapses to maps. Annu Rev Neurosci 1998;21:149-86.

[80] Hodzic A, Veit R, Karim AA, Erb M, Godde B. Improvement and decline in tactile discrimination behavior after cortical plasticity induced by passive tactile coactivation. J Neurosci 2004;24(2):442-6.

[81] Jenkins WM, Merzenich MM, Ochs MT, Allard T, Guic-Robles E. Functional reorganization of primary somatosensory cortex in adult owl monkeys after behaviorally controlled tactile stimulation. J Neurophysiol 1990;63(1):82-104.

[82] Rauschecker JP. Mechanisms of visual plasticity: Hebb synapses, NMDA receptors, and beyond. Physiol Rev 1991;71(2):587-615.

[83] Hebb D. The organization of behavior. New York: Wiley, 1949.

[84] Inan M, Crair MC. Development of cortical maps: perspectives from the barrel cortex. Neuroscientist 2007;13(1):49-61.

[85] Fernandez-de-las-Penas C, de la Llave-Rincon AI, Fernandez-Carnero J, Cuadrado ML, Arendt-Nielsen L, Pareja JA. Bilateral widespread mechanical pain sensitivity in carpal tunnel syndrome: evidence of central processing in unilateral neuropathy. Brain 2009;132(Pt 6):1472-9.

[86] Fernandez-de-Las-Penas C, Madeleine P, Martinez-Perez A, Arendt-Nielsen L, Jimenez-Garcia R, Pareja JA. Pressure pain sensitivity topographical maps reveal bilateral hyperalgesia of the hands in patients with unilateral carpal tunnel syndrome. Arthritis Care Res (Hoboken) 2010;62(8):1055-64.

[87] de la Llave-Rincon AI, Fernandez-de-las-Penas C, Fernandez-Carnero J, Padua L, Arendt-Nielsen L, Pareja JA. Bilateral hand/wrist heat and cold hyperalgesia, but not hypoesthesia, in unilateral carpal tunnel syndrome. Exp Brain Res 2009;198(4):455-63.

[88] Zanette G, Marani S, Tamburin S. Extra-median spread of sensory symptoms in carpal tunnel syndrome suggests the presence of pain-related mechanisms. Pain 2006;122(3):264-70.

[89] Zanette G, Cacciatori C, Tamburin S. Central sensitization in carpal tunnel syndrome with extraterritorial spread of sensory symptoms. Pain 2010;148(2):227-36.

[90] Apkarian AV, Sosa Y, Sonty S, Levy RM, Harden RN, Parrish TB, et al. Chronic back pain is associated with decreased prefrontal and thalamic gray matter density. J Neurosci 2004;24(46):10410-5.

[91] Flor H, Braun C, Elbert T, Birbaumer N. Extensive reorganization of primary somatosensory cortex in chronic back pain patients. Neurosci Lett 1997;224(1):5-8.

[92] Juottonen K, Gockel M, Silen T, Hurri H, Hari R, Forss N. Altered central sensorimotor processing in patients with complex regional pain syndrome. Pain 2002;98(3):315-23.

[93] Maihofner C, Handwerker HO, Neundorfer B, Birklein F. Patterns of cortical reorganization in complex regional pain syndrome. Neurology 2003;61(12):1707-15.

[94] Tamburin S, Cacciatori C, Marani S, Zanette G. Pain and motor function in carpal tunnel syndrome: a clinical, neurophysiological and psychophysical study. J Neurol 2008;255(11):1636-43.

[95] Jeng OJ, Radwin RG, Fryback DG. Preliminary evaluation of a sensory and psychomotor functional test battery for carpal tunnel syndrome: Part 1--Confirmed cases and normal subjects. Am Ind Hyg Assoc J 1997;58(12):852-60.

[96] Huisstede BM, Randsdorp MS, Coert JH, Glerum S, van Middelkoop M, Koes BW. Carpal tunnel syndrome. Part II: effectiveness of surgical treatments--a systematic review. Arch Phys Med Rehabil 2010;91(7):1005-24.

[97] Huisstede BM, Hoogvliet P, Randsdorp MS, Glerum S, van Middelkoop M, Koes BW. Carpal tunnel syndrome. Part I: effectiveness of nonsurgical treatments--a systematic review. Arch Phys Med Rehabil 2010;91(7):981-1004.

[98] Weber RA, DeSalvo DJ, Rude MJ. Five-year follow-up of carpal tunnel release in patients over age 65. J Hand Surg Am 2010;35(2):207-11.

[99]   Radwin RG, Sesto ME, Zachary SV. Functional tests to quantify recovery following carpal tunnel release. J Bone Joint Surg Am 2004;86-A(12):2614-20.

[100] Hsu HY, Kuo LC, Chiu HY, Jou IM, Su FC. Functional sensibility assessment. Part II: Effects of sensory improvement on precise pinch force modulation after transverse carpal tunnel release. J Orthop Res 2009;27(11):1534-9.

[101] Povlsen B, Tegnell I. Incidence and natural history of touch allodynia after open carpal tunnel release. Scand J Plast Reconstr Surg Hand Surg 1996;30(3):221-5.

[102] Boya H, Ozcan O, Oztekin HH. Long-term complications of open carpal tunnel release. Muscle Nerve 2008;38(5):1443-6.

[103] Taylor KS, Anastakis DJ, Davis KD. Chronic pain and sensorimotor deficits following peripheral nerve injury. Pain 2010 Jul 22.

[104] Kuo MH, Leong CP, Cheng YF, Chang HW. Static wrist position associated with least median nerve compression: sonographic evaluation. Am J Phys Med Rehabil 2001;80(4):256-60.

[105] Burke DT, Burke MM, Stewart GW, Cambre A. Splinting for carpal tunnel syndrome: in search of the optimal angle. Arch Phys Med Rehabil 1994;75(11):1241-4.

[106] Manente G, Torrieri F, Di Blasio F, Staniscia T, Romano F, Uncini A. An innovative hand brace for carpal tunnel syndrome: a randomized controlled trial. Muscle Nerve 2001;24(8):1020-5.

[107] De Angelis MV, Pierfelice F, Di Giovanni P, Staniscia T, Uncini A. Efficacy of a soft hand brace and a wrist splint for carpal tunnel syndrome: a randomized controlled study. Acta Neurol Scand 2009;119(1):68-74.

[108] Ucan H, Yagci I, Yilmaz L, Yagmurlu F, Keskin D, Bodur H. Comparison of splinting, splinting plus local steroid injection and open carpal tunnel release outcomes in idiopathic carpal tunnel syndrome. Rheumatol Int 2006;27(1):45-51.

[109] Sevim S, Dogu O, Camdeviren H, Kaleagasi H, Aral M, Arslan E, et al. Long-term effectiveness of steroid injections and splinting in mild and moderate carpal tunnel syndrome. Neurol Sci 2004;25(2):48-52.

[110] Armstrong T, Devor W, Borschel L, Contreras R. Intracarpal steroid injection is safe and effective for short-term management of carpal tunnel syndrome. Muscle Nerve 2004;29(1):82-8.

[111] Agarwal V, Singh R, Sachdev A, Wiclaff, Shekhar S, Goel D. A prospective study of the long-term efficacy of local methyl prednisolone acetate injection in the management of mild carpal tunnel syndrome. Rheumatology (Oxford) 2005;44(5):647-50.

[112] Celiker R, Arslan S, Inanici F. Corticosteroid injection vs. nonsteroidal antiinflammatory drug and splinting in carpal tunnel syndrome. Am J Phys Med Rehabil 2002;81(3):182-6.

[113] Cherng CH, Wong CS, Ho ST. Spinal actions of nonsteroidal anti-inflammatory drugs. Acta Anaesthesiol Sin 1996;34(2):81-8.

[114] Sim H, Shin BC, Lee MS, Jung A, Lee H, Ernst E. Acupuncture for carpal tunnel syndrome: A systematic review of randomized controlled trials. J Pain 2010 Nov 17.

Neuroplasticity in carpal tunnel syndrome 179

[115] Naeser MA, Hahn KA, Lieberman BE, Branco KF. Carpal tunnel syndrome pain treated with low-level laser and microamperes transcutaneous electric nerve stimulation: A controlled study. Arch Phys Med Rehabil 2002;83(7):978-88.

[116] Chen G. The effect of acupuncture treatment on carpal tunnel syndrome. Am J Acupuncture 1990;19(1):5-9.

[117] Gelnar PA, Krauss BR, Szeverenyi NM, Apkarian AV. Fingertip representation in the human somatosensory cortex: an fMRI study. Neuroimage 1998;7(4 Pt 1):261-83.

[118] Kurth R, Villringer K, Mackert BM, Schwiemann J, Braun J, Curio G, et al. fMRI assessment of somatotopy in human Brodmann area 3b by electrical finger stimulation. Neuroreport 1998;9(2):207-12.

[119] McGlone F, Kelly EF, Trulsson M, Francis ST, Westling G, Bowtell R. Functional neuroimaging studies of human somatosensory cortex. Behav Brain Res 2002;135(1-2):147-58.

[120] Kara M, Ozcakar L, Gokcay D, Ozcelik E, Yorubulut M, Guneri S, et al. Quantification of the effects of transcutaneous electrical nerve stimulation with functional magnetic resonance imaging: a double-blind randomized placebo-controlled study. Arch Phys Med Rehabil 2010;91(8):1160-5.

[121] Sandberg M, Lundeberg T, Lindberg LG, Gerdle B. Effects of acupuncture on skin and muscle blood flow in healthy subjects. Eur J Appl Physiol 2003;90(1-2):114-9.

[122] Andersson S, Lundeberg T. Acupuncture - from empiricism to science: functional background to acupuncture effects in pain and disease. Med Hypotheses 1995;45:271-81.

[123] Lundeberg T. Peripheral effects of sensory nerve stimulation (acupuncture) in inflammation and ischemia. Scand J Rehabil Med Suppl 1993;29:61-86.

[124] Sato A, Sato Y, Shimura M, Uchida S. Calcitonin gene-related peptide produces skeletal muscle vasodilation following antidromic stimulation of unmyelinated afferents in the dorsal root in rats. Neurosci Lett 2000;283(2):137-40.

[125] Hui K, Liu J, Rosen B, Kwong K. Effects of acupuncture on human limbic system and basal ganglia measured by fMRI. Neuroimage 1997;5(4):s226.

[126] Hui KK, Liu J, Makris N, Gollub RL, Chen AJ, Moore CI, et al. Acupuncture modulates the limbic system and subcortical gray structures of the human brain: evidence from fMRI studies in normal subjects. Hum Brain Mapp 2000;9(1):13-25.

[127] Napadow V, Makris N, Liu J, Kettner NW, Kwong KK, Hui KK. Effects of electroacupuncture versus manual acupuncture on the human brain as measured by fMRI. Hum Brain Mapp 2005;24(3):193-205.

[128] Wu MT, Xiong J, Yang PC, Hsieh JC, Tsai G, Cheng HM, et al. Central processing of acupuncture in human brain evaluated by functional mr imaging. Proceed Int Society Magnetic Resonance Med, 1997:723.

[129] Kandel E, Schwartz J, Jessell T. Principles of neural science. 4th ed. New York: McGraw Hill, 2000.

[130] Bernard J, GE H, JM B. Nucleus centralis of the amygdala and the globus pallida ventralis. Electrophysiological evidence for an involvement in pain processes. J Neruophysiol 1992;68(551-69).

[131] Willis WD, Westlund KN. Neuroanatomy of the pain system and of the pathways that modulate pain. J Clin Neurophysiol 1997;14(1):2-31.

[132] Amaral D, Price J, Pitkanen A, Carmichael S. Anatomical organization of the primate amygdaloid complex. In: Aggleton J, editor. The amygdala: Neurobiological aspects of emotion, memory, and mental dysfunction. New York: Wiley-Liss, 1992:1-66.

[133] Zald DH. The human amygdala and the emotional evaluation of sensory stimuli. Brain Res Brain Res Rev 2003;41(1):88-123.

[134] Parent A. Carpenter's human neuroanatomy, 9th ed. Baltimore, MD: Williams Wilkins, 1996.

[135] Lang PJ, Bradley MM, Fitzsimmons JR, Cuthbert BN, Scott JD, Moulder B, et al. Emotional arousal and activation of the visual cortex: an fMRI analysis. Psychophysiology 1998;35(2):199-210.

[136] Quirk GJ, Armony JL, LeDoux JE. Fear conditioning enhances different temporal components of tone-evoked spike trains in auditory cortex and lateral amygdala. Neuron 1997;19(3):613-24.

[137] Zhang WT, Jin Z, Cui GH, Zhang KL, Zhang L, Zeng YW, et al. Relations between brain network activation and analgesic effect induced by low vs. high frequency electrical acupoint stimulation in different subjects: a functional magnetic resonance imaging study. Brain Res 2003;982(2):168-78.

[138] Jacobs S, Anderson G, Bailey S, Ottaviano J, McCarthy V. Neurophysiological correlates of acupuncture: limbic and thalamic responses to analgesic studies in non-human primates. TIT J Life Sci 1977;7(3-4):37-42.

[139] Napadow V, Kettner N, Liu J, Li M, Kwong KK, Vangel M, et al. Hypothalamus and amygdala response to acupuncture stimuli in carpal tunnel syndrome. Pain 2007;130(3):254-66.

[140] Letzkus JJ, Kampa BM, Stuart GJ. Does spike timing-dependent synaptic plasticity underlie memory formation? Clin Exp Pharmacol Physiol 2007;34(10):1070-6.

[141] Pfister JP, Tass PA. STDP in oscillatory recurrent networks: Theoretical conditions for desynchronization and applications to deep brain stimulation. Front Comput Neurosci 2010;4.

[142] Hauck M, Lorenz J, Engel AK. Role of synchronized oscillatory brain activity for human pain perception. Rev Neurosci 2008;19(6):441-50.

[143] Warren CP, Hu S, Stead M, Brinkmann BH, Bower MR, Worrell GA. Synchrony in normal and focal epileptic brain: The seizure onset zone is functionally disconnected. J Neurophysiol 2010 Oct 6.

[144] Hauptmann C, Tass PA. Therapeutic rewiring by means of desynchronizing brain stimulation. Biosystems 2007;89(1-3):173-81.

[145] Hauptmann C, Tass PA. Restoration of segregated, physiological neuronal connectivity by desynchronizing stimulation. J Neural Eng 2010;7(5):056008.

[146] Rosen B, Bjorkman A, Weibull A, Svensson J, Lundborg G. Improved sensibility of the foot after temporary cutaneous anesthesia of the lower leg. Neuroreport 2009;20(1):37-41.

[147] Lundborg GN, Bjorkman AC, Rosen BN, Nilsson JA, Dahlin LB. Cutaneous anaesthesia of the lower leg can improve sensibility in the diabetic foot. A double-blind, randomized clinical trial. Diabet Med 2010;27(7):823-9.

[148] Lissek S, Wilimzig C, Stude P, Pleger B, Kalisch T, Maier C, et al. Immobilization impairs tactile perception and shrinks somatosensory cortical maps. Curr Biol 2009;19(10):837-42.

Acknowledgments

Chapter X

About the editors

Helena Knotkova, PhD is Co-Chief of the Research Division, Department of Pain Medicine and Palliative Care, Beth Israel Medical Center, New York, Director of Research, Institute of Non-invasive Brain Stimulation of New York in the same institution, and Assistant Professor of Neurology, Albert Einstein College of Medicine, Bronx, New York. She received her degrees in psychology (Doctor of Philosophy from Charles' University, Prague) and in biological sciences (PhD) from the Department of Cellular Neurophysiology, Institute of Physiology, Czech Academy of Sciences, Prague. Her background and training have enabled Dr. Knotkova to adopt a multi-disciplinary approach to the study of patho-physiological mechanisms of pain and facilitated her research and implementation of novel treatment strategies in pain management, including tDCS. In addition to being a member of the International Association for the Study of Pain since 1995 and American Pain Society since 2000, she also serves as a Section Editor for the Journal of Pain Management (JPM), a member of the Editorial Board of the Open Pain Journal and she serves as a reviewer for various medical journals. She has served as Guest Editor of the Special Issue of JPM on Brain Stimulation, and Editor of the book Brain Stimulation for the Treatment of Pain, and authored and co-authored numerous peer reviewed publications, chapters and presentations at international meetings. E-mail: HKnotkov@chpnet.org

Ricardo A Cruciani, MD, PhD is Vice-Chairman and Chief of the Pain Medicine Division in the Department of Pain Medicine and Palliative Care at Beth Israel Medical Center, New York, Director of the Institute for Non-Invasive Brain Stimulation in the same institution and Associate Professor in the Department of Neurology at Albert Einstein College of

Medicine, Bronx, New York. He attended the University of Buenos Aires, School of Medicine, where he received his MD degree and a PhD degree in Pharmacology (Suma Cum Laude). After working in basic neuroscience at the National Institutes of Health for almost a decade, he completed a residency program at Weill Medical College of Cornell University in Neurology and Psychiatry and received postgraduate training in Pain Management and Palliative Care at Memorial Sloan Kettering Cancer Center, New York. He has published more than one hundred publications including peer reviewed journals, book chapters and editorials. He has lectured nationally and internationally and has numerous presentations at scientific meetings. In addition he served in the Program Committee and the Nomination Committee of the American pain Society whre he is now a member of the Board of Directors. He was the Editor in Chief of the journal Advances in Pain Medicine. He serves in the editorial board of the Journal of Pauin and Symptom Management and is an ad hoc reviewer in numerous journals including the journals Anesthesia and Analgesia, Neurology and The Journal of Physiology, He also participated at NIH study sections and has been an NIH grantee for several years. E-mail: rcrucian@bethisraelny.org

Joav Merrick, MD, MMedSci, DMSc, is professor of pediatrics, child health and human development affiliated with Kentucky Children's Hospital, University of Kentucky, Lexington, United States, the medical director of the Health Services, Division for Mental Retardation, Ministry of Social Affairs, Jerusalem, the founder and director of the National Institute of Child Health and Human Development, Jerusalem, Israel. Numerous publications in the field of pediatrics, child health and human development, rehabilitation, intellectual disability, disability, health, welfare, abuse, advocacy, quality of life and prevention. Received the Peter Sabroe Child Award for outstanding work on behalf of Danish Children in 1985 and the International LEGO-Prize ("The Children's Nobel Prize") for an extraordinary contribution towards improvement in child welfare and well-being in 1987. E-mail: jmerrick@zahav.net.il

Chapter XI

About the Institute for Noninvasive Brain Stimulation of New York

The Institute for Noninvasive Brain Stimulation of New York was established in 2008 within the Department of Pain Medicine and Palliative Care, Beth Israel Medical Center, New York (website: http://www.stoppain.org/). Since then, we have conducted hundreds of tDCS sessions in patients with various chronic pain syndromes including:

- Pain Complex Regional Syndrome, formerly known as Reflex Sympathetic Dystrophy (CRPS/RSD)
- Fibromyalgia
- Migraines
- Phantom-limb Pain
- Post-Stroke Pain Syndrome
- Low-back Pain
- Trigeminal Neuralgia and other types of facial pain

Our mission is to provide non-invasive techniques (e.g. Transcranial Direct Current Stimulation, tDCS), to relieve chronic pain in patients, whose pain does not respond to conventional therapies.

The Institute for Non-invasive Brain Stimulation of New York is an integral part of the Department of Pain Medicine and Palliative Care, Beth Israel Medical Center, which offers a broad array of therapies for chronic pain of all types.

The highly trained medical team of the Department includes pain specialists with backgrounds in Neurology, Rehabilitation Medicine, Anesthesiology, and Psychology. During its 10 year history, the Department has received numerous awards; the most recently, a "2009 Center of Excellence" award by the American Pain Society.

Contact: Ricardo Cruciani, MD, PhD
Director, Institute for Noninvasive Brain Stimulation
Department of Pain Medicine and Palliative Care
350 East 17th Street, Baird Hall, 12th floor
Beth Israel Medical Center
New York, NY 10003
United States
E-mail: rcrucian@bethisraelny.org

Chapter XII

About the National Institute of Child Health and Human Development in Israel

The National Institute of Child Health and Human Development (NICHD) in Israel was established in 1998 as a virtual institute under the auspicies of the Medical Director, Ministry of Social Affairs and Social Services in order to function as the research arm for the Office of the Medical Director. In 1998 the National Council for Child Health and Pediatrics, Ministry of Health and in 1999 the Director General and Deputy Director General of the Ministry of Health endorsed the establishment of the NICHD.

Mission

The mission of a National Institute for Child Health and Human Development in Israel is to provide an academic focal point for the scholarly interdisciplinary study of child life, health, public health, welfare, disability, rehabilitation, intellectual disability and related aspects of human development. This mission includes research, teaching, clinical work, information and public service activities in the field of child health and human development.

Service and academic activities

Over the years many activities became focused in the south of Israel due to collaboration with various professionals at the Faculty of Health Sciences (FOHS) at the Ben Gurion University of the Negev (BGU). Since 2000 an affiliation with the Zusman Child Development Center at the Pediatric Division of Soroka University Medical Center has resulted in collaboration around the establishment of the Down Syndrome Clinic at that center. In 2002 a full course on "Disability" was established at the Recanati School for Allied Professions in the Community, FOHS, BGU and in 2005 collaboration was started with the Primary Care Unit of the faculty and disability became part of the master of public health course on "Children and society". In the academic year 2005-2006 a one semester course on "Aging with disability" was started as part of the master of science program in gerontology in our collaboration with the Center for Multidisciplinary Research in Aging.

Research activities

The affiliated staff have over the years published work from projects and research activities in this national and international collaboration. In the year 2000 the International Journal of Adolescent Medicine and Health and in 2005 the International Journal on Disability and Human development of Freund Publishing House (London and Tel Aviv), in the year 2003 the TSW-Child Health and Human Development and in 2006 the TSW-Holistic Health and Medicine of the Scientific World Journal (New York and Kirkkonummi, Finland), all peer-reviewed international journals were affiliated with the National Institute of Child Health and Human Development. From 2008 also the International Journal of Child Health and Human Development (Nova Science, New York), the International Journal of Child and Adolescent Health (Nova Science) and the Journal of Pain Management (Nova Science) affiliated and from 2009 the International Public Health Journal (Nova Science) and Journal of Alternative Medicine Research (Nova Science).

National collaborations

Nationally the NICHD works in collaboration with the Faculty of Health Sciences, Ben Gurion University of the Negev; Department of Physical

Therapy, Sackler School of Medicine, Tel Aviv University; Autism Center, Assaf HaRofeh Medical Center; National Rett and PKU Centers at Chaim Sheba Medical Center, Tel HaShomer; Department of Physiotherapy, Haifa University; Department of Education, Bar Ilan University, Ramat Gan, Faculty of Social Sciences and Health Sciences; College of Judea and Samaria in Ariel and in 2011 NICHD became affiliated with the Department of Pediatrics, Mt Scopus Campus, Hebrew University Hadassah Medical Center in Jerusalem.

International collaborations

Internationally with the Department of Disability and Human Development, College of Applied Health Sciences, University of Illinois at Chicago; Strong Center for Developmental Disabilities, Golisano Children's Hospital at Strong, University of Rochester School of Medicine and Dentistry, New York; Centre on Intellectual Disabilities, University of Albany, New York; Centre for Chronic Disease Prevention and Control, Health Canada, Ottawa; Chandler Medical Center and Children's Hospital, Kentucky Children's Hospital, Section of Adolescent Medicine, University of Kentucky, Lexington; Chronic Disease Prevention and Control Research Center, Baylor College of Medicine, Houston, Texas; Division of Neuroscience, Department of Psychiatry, Columbia University, New York; Institute for the Study of Disadvantage and Disability, Atlanta; Center for Autism and Related Disorders, Department Psychiatry, Children's Hospital Boston, Boston; Department of Paediatrics, Child Health and Adolescent Medicine, Children's Hospital at Westmead, Westmead, Australia; International Centre for the Study of Occupational and Mental Health, Düsseldorf, Germany; Centre for Advanced Studies in Nursing, Department of General Practice and Primary Care, University of Aberdeen, Aberdeen, United Kingdom; Quality of Life Research Center, Copenhagen, Denmark; Nordic School of Public Health, Gottenburg, Sweden; Scandinavian Institute of Quality of Working Life, Oslo, Norway; Centre for Quality of Life of the Hong Kong Institute of Asia-Pacific Studies and School of Social Work, Chinese University, Hong Kong.

Targets

Our focus is on research, international collaborations, clinical work, teaching and policy in health, disability and human development and to establish the NICHD as a permanent institute at one of the residential care centers for persons with intellectual disability in Israel in order to conduct model research and together with the four university schools of public health/medicine in Israel establish a national master and doctoral program in disability and human development at the institute to secure the next generation of professionals working in this often non-prestigious/low-status field of work. For this project we need your support. We are looking for all kinds of support and eventually an endowment.

Contact: Joav Merrick, MD, DMSc
Professor of Pediatrics, Child Health and Human Development
Medical Director, Division for Mental Retardation,
Ministry of Social Affairs and Social Services,
POB 1260, IL-91012 Jerusalem, Israel.
E-mail: jmerrick@inter.net.il

Chapter XIII

About the disability studies book series

Disability studies is a book series with publications from a multidisciplinary group of researchers, practitioners and clinicians for an international professional forum interested in the broad spectrum of disability, intellectual disability, health and human development.

- Reiter S. Disability from a humanistic perspective: Towards a better quality of life. New York: Nova Science, 2008
- Knotkova H, Cruciani R, Merrick J, eds. Pain. Brain stimulation in the treatment of pain. New York: Nova Science, 2010.
- Prasher VP, ed. Contemporary issues in intellectual disabilities. New York: Nova Science, 2010.
- Lotan M, Merrick J, eds. Rett syndrome: Therapeutic interventions. New York: Nova Science, 2011.
- Satgé D, Merrick J, eds. Cancer in children and adults with intellectual disabilities: Current research aspects. New York: Nova Science, 2011.

Contact: Professor Joav Merrick, MD, MMedSci, DMSc
Medical Director, Division for Mental Retardation
Ministry of Social Affairs and Social Serives
POBox 1260
IL-91012 Jerusalem, Israel
E-mail: jmerrick@zahav.net.il

Index

A

abatement, 164
abuse, 186
accelerator, 102
access, 2, 118, 176
acetaminophen, 12, 17, 18, 28
acid, 7, 11, 12, 16, 22, 53, 54, 60, 111, 161
acidosis, 7
acromegaly, 154
action potential, 7, 42, 49, 51, 54, 62, 169
acupuncture, 62, 154, 156, 166, 167, 168, 169, 170, 173, 179, 180
adaptation, 78, 92, 93, 117
ADC, 158
adenosine, 8, 52, 58, 59
adenosine triphosphate, 8, 59
adjustment, 97, 143
adulthood, 93
adults, 44, 162, 168, 170, 193
advancement, 16
adverse effects, 2, 4, 20, 23, 140
adverse event, 141, 167
advocacy, 186
affective dimension, 74, 75, 76
affective disorder, 125
affective experience, 70
age, 2, 108, 109, 112, 124, 125, 155, 177
agonist, 18, 26, 27, 28, 53, 62, 81
alcohol use, 165

allergic rhinitis, 5
alters, 17, 30, 84, 175
amino, 53
amino acid, 53
amplitude, 104
amputation, 79, 80, 81, 86, 87, 94, 95, 100, 104, 142, 149, 150, 160, 176
amygdala, 73, 76, 119, 168, 179, 180
amyloidosis, 154
analgesic, 2, 3, 4, 7, 10, 12, 13, 16, 17, 21, 22, 27, 28, 30, 31, 61, 62, 65, 72, 76, 133, 140, 144, 146, 148, 151, 180
analgesic agent, 12, 13, 21, 22
anatomy, 75, 105, 117
anisotropy, 158
anorexia, 171
antagonism, 11
anterior cingulate cortex, 65, 74, 75, 119, 122
antibody, 11, 28, 61
antidepressants, 62, 73, 76, 135
anti-inflammatory drugs, 178
antipyretic, 17, 18
antisense, 11, 24
antisense oligonucleotides, 11, 24
anxiety, 73, 111, 117, 128
anxiety disorder, 73
aphasia, 140
apoptosis, 57, 159, 175
arousal, 74, 79, 180

Index

arrest, 139, 141, 142
artery, 109
arthritis, 38
Asia, 191
aspartate, 53, 64, 66, 81, 110, 127, 161
assessment, 20, 123, 124, 174, 178, 179
asthma, 7, 25
astrocytes, 38, 40, 44, 48, 56, 58, 59
asymptomatic, 138, 141
ATP, 8, 9, 26, 40, 58, 59, 61
atrophy, 117, 155
atypical methylxanthine, 41
auditory cortex, 86, 119, 180
autoimmune diseases, 67
autoimmunity, 67
avoidance, 119
awareness, 75, 81, 88
axonal degeneration, 159
axonal pathology, 158
axons, 52, 64, 158, 173

B

back pain, 78, 82, 84, 86, 89, 111, 117, 125, 127, 128, 148, 154, 164, 177
basal ganglia, 104, 133, 179
base, 135, 141
behavioral disorders, 169
behaviors, 44, 83, 173
beneficial effect, 78, 85
benefits, 85, 108, 115, 143, 148
biofeedback, 72, 75
biological sciences, 185
biomechanics, 164
blood, 40, 58, 71, 86, 109, 110, 167, 179
blood flow, 71, 86, 110, 167, 179
blood vessels, 40
BMA, 28
body image, 82, 89
body schema, 83, 89, 101
bone, 10, 16, 31, 40, 156, 165
bone cancer, 10, 16, 31
bone marrow, 40
brachial plexus, 142, 144, 146
bradykinin, 8, 9, 55

brain, xiii, xix, xx, 18, 28, 40, 44, 45, 47, 48, 52, 55, 58, 62, 65, 66, 69, 70, 71, 72, 74, 75, 76, 78, 79, 82, 83, 84, 85, 86, 90, 92, 93, 95, 96, 97, 98, 99, 101, 102, 103, 106, 107, 110, 111, 112, 115, 121, 122, 125, 126, 127, 128, 132, 133, 134, 135, 136, 143, 144, 147, 148, 150, 152, 154, 156, 160, 164, 165, 167, 168, 169, 170, 180
brain activity, 110, 170, 180
brain damage, 86
brain functioning, 165
brain structure, 52, 69, 71, 72, 168
brainstem, 52, 72, 93, 141, 142, 144, 160
Brazil, 123
Britain, 28
Buddhism, 100
bunionectomy, 5, 14
burn, 44

C

calcitonin, 7, 37, 49, 167
calcitonin gene-regulated peptide (CGRP), 167
calcium, 12, 15, 38, 41, 53, 54, 60
cancer, 2, 17
candidates, 22, 144
capsaicin concentration patches, 22
carboxylic acid, 30
carpal tunnel release, 155, 164, 165, 172, 173, 177, 178
carpal tunnel syndrome(CTS), xii, 153, 154, 171, 172, 173, 174, 175, 177, 178, 179, 180
case studies, 89
catheter, 159
cation, 25
CCA, 149
central nervous system (CNS), 18, 24, 28, 31, 35, 37, 38, 40, 41, 43, 44, 48, 52, 53, 54, 58, 59, 62, 63, 70, 73, 92, 103, 108, 110, 153, 154, 165, 166, 168, 169
cerebellum, 98, 99, 102
cerebral blood flow, 71

Index

cerebral cortex, 104, 126, 175
cerebral hemisphere, 119
challenges, 93, 110, 123
channel blocker, 41
chemical, 3, 7, 12, 18, 48, 49, 52, 56, 59, 110
chemicals, 36
chemokine receptor, 40, 59, 67
chemokines, 48, 49, 58, 59
Chicago, 123, 124, 191
children, 193
chinese medicine, 13
CHO cells, 12
cholecystectomy, 14
choline, 110
cigarette smoking, 155
circulation, 22
classification, 134, 136, 150, 172
cleavage, 40, 45
clinical application, xx, 27, 125
clinical problems, 117
clinical trials, 2, 3, 4, 5, 13, 20, 22, 23, 32, 60, 61, 63
clone, 4
cloning, 4, 16, 21, 24
cluster headache, 14, 29, 127
cocaine, 127
coding, 126, 127
coffee, 19
cognition, 163, 169
cognitive psychology, 96
cognitive research, 125
cognitive system, xx, 169
cognitive tasks, 105
coherence, 162, 163
collaboration, 190
collagen, 160
collateral, 56, 60
common findings, 34
communication, 169
community, 44, 173
comorbidity, 73
compensation, 171
complex regional pain syndrome (CRPS), 79, 87, 100

complexity, xv, xvi, 38, 43
compliance, 13, 22
complications, 124, 178
composition, 71, 117
compounds, 2, 3, 5, 22, 60, 61, 62
compression, 109, 154, 155, 156, 157, 158, 159, 163, 166, 169, 172, 173, 175, 178
computed tomography, 71
computer, 71, 102, 103
conditioning, 168, 169, 180
conductance, 54, 57
conduction, 7, 155, 157, 158, 160, 161, 162, 166, 167, 172, 174, 175
conference, 155
conflict, 123
congress, 125
congruence, 96
connective tissue, 159, 174, 175
connectivity, 72, 78, 97, 99, 160, 180
consensus, 155
consumption, 14, 21, 147
control group, 15, 21, 114, 120
controlled studies, 147
controlled trials, 132, 178
coordination, 83, 155
coping strategies, 72
corpus callosum, 117
correlation, 124, 146, 150, 152
correlations, 123, 155
cortex, 7, 48, 62, 70, 71, 72, 73, 74, 75, 78, 79, 80, 81, 82, 84, 86, 87, 88, 89, 90, 93, 95, 96, 97, 98, 99, 102, 103, 104, 105, 106, 111, 112, 113, 114, 115, 116, 117, 118, 119, 120, 121, 122, 126, 127, 128, 132, 135, 140, 144, 146, 148, 149, 150, 151, 152, 154, 156, 160, 161, 162, 167, 168, 176, 177, 179, 180
cortical neurons, 80, 93
cortical pathway, 96, 168
cortical systems, 93, 122
corticosteroids, 154
cost, 154
cough, 13, 20
covering, 114
craniotomy, 140

creatine, 110
cross-sectional study, 154
cues, 76, 127
culture, 100
cure, 22
cycling, 135, 156, 157
cytoarchitecture, 117
cytokines, 40, 43, 46, 48, 49, 56, 58, 59, 60, 65
cytotoxicity, 6

D

daily living, 99
damages, 157
damping, 97
dance, 95
data set, 102
database, 3, 124
deep brain stimulation(DBS), 132, 133, 136, 137, 150, 170, 180
degradation, 79
dehiscence, 138, 141
Delta, 64
demyelination, 67, 109, 175
dendrites, 40
dendritic spines, 45
Denmark, 191
Department of Education, 191
dephosphorylation, 9
depolarization, 26, 38, 53, 54, 56, 57
depression, 62, 73, 76, 78, 117, 127
depressive symptoms, 86
deprivation, 94
desensitization, 2, 4, 7, 9, 10, 13, 22, 23, 27
desynchronization, 180
detection, 19, 23, 72, 84, 90, 110, 143, 165
diabetes, 154, 170
diabetic neuropathy, 1, 13, 15, 66, 170
diffusion, 125, 158, 174
disability, xii, 100, 186, 189, 190, 192, 193
discrimination, 80, 82, 86, 87, 88, 142, 143, 165, 166, 176
discrimination learning, 88
discrimination training, 80, 86, 87

disorder, 107, 108, 112
displacement, 79
distribution, 45, 71, 76, 110, 124, 134, 135
diversity, 26
dogs, 19
DOI, 151
dopamine, 7
dorsal horn, 31, 39, 44, 47, 48, 64, 65, 66, 70, 159
dorsolateral prefrontal cortex, 84, 111, 115, 117, 164
dosing, 18, 19
double blind study, 170
drug addict, 44
drug discovery, 24
drug targets, 64, 73
drug treatment, 76
drugs, 2, 4, 7, 17, 22, 23, 27, 62, 135
Dublin Free Press, 3, 23
durability, 156, 165
dysarthria, 142
dysphagia, 143
dystonia, 89, 94, 104

E

edema, 7, 156, 157, 159
editors, xii, 89, 172, 185
elderly population, 109
electrodes, 80, 168
electroencephalography, 170
electromagnetic, 133
electromyography, 172
elucidation, 23
EMG, 98, 174
emotion, xv, 70, 72, 75, 92, 117, 119, 128, 180
emotional experience, 48
emotional responses, 72, 111
emotional state, 71
encoding, xv, 11, 169
endorphins, 52
endothelial cells, 159
endotoxins, 17
England, 86

Index

enkephalins, 52
enlargement, 79, 80, 94, 171
entorhinal cortex, 119
entrapment, 153, 154, 170
environment, 17, 83
environmental change, 40
environmental stimuli, 100
epidemiologic studies, 172
epidemiology, 124
epidural hematoma, 138, 140, 141
epilepsy, 93, 141, 142, 169
episodic memory, 98
episodic memory tasks, 98
ester, 30
estrogen, 158, 174
ethanol, 8
etiology, 160
Europe, 3, 14
European Community, 85
everyday life, 95
evidence, xx, 10, 15, 21, 23, 40, 63, 72, 75,
  81, 82, 84, 86, 88, 96, 99, 104, 106, 126,
  132, 134, 144, 147, 155, 156, 159, 160,
  165, 166, 170, 175, 177, 179
evoked potential, 127, 148, 160
evolution, 169, 171
excitability, 36, 38, 44, 52, 53, 57, 58, 78,
  84, 93, 95, 96, 104, 105, 126, 132, 133,
  134
excitation, 7, 26
excitatory synapses, 38
execution, 98, 105, 164
executive function, 117
exercise, 100, 102
exposure, 10, 36, 168
extensor, 96
external influences, 93
extraction, 3, 18, 20, 21, 116, 127, 142

F

facial pain, xii, 123, 124, 131, 132, 134,
  135, 136, 140, 141, 142, 144, 146, 147,
  148, 150, 151, 187
false negative, 158

fat, 158
fear, 22, 70, 73, 111, 119
feelings, 100, 111
fever, 13
fiber, 39, 42, 121, 122, 158
fibers, xx, 7, 34, 35, 37, 41, 42, 49, 50, 52,
  55, 56, 114, 115, 121, 122, 128, 158
fibromyalgia, 12, 62, 66, 75, 82, 84, 86, 89,
  90, 95, 104, 111, 115, 125, 127, 133, 149
fibrosis, 156, 157, 158, 159, 160
Finland, 190
flavor, 2
flexor, 96, 155, 174
fluid, 158
focal seizure, 141
food, 2, 28
food intake, 28
force, 46, 99, 178
formation, 7, 162
free radicals, 156
freedom, 155, 164
frontal cortex, 111, 115, 116
functional changes, 111, 115, 126, 132, 135,
  150, 153, 154
functional imaging, 71, 72, 104, 128, 171
functional MRI, 75, 128, 154
funding, 85, 123, 171
fusion, 160

G

gait, 97
gamma rays, 71
Gamma-aminobutyric acid (GABA), 12, 51,
  54, 57, 59, 62, 65, 111, 161, 176
ganglion, 45, 65, 112, 126
gastroesophageal reflux, 21
gender differences, 158
gene expression, 155
gene therapy, 67
gene transfer, 62, 67
generalized seizures, 138
genetic blueprint, 93
geometry, 158
Germany, 77, 131, 191

200 Index

gerontology, 190
ginger, 8
GlaxoSmithKline, 16, 19, 20
glia, 40, 43, 46, 57, 58, 65, 66
glial cells, 40, 41, 48, 58
globus, 179
glossopharyngeal nerve, 141
glutamate, 16, 31, 37, 38, 49, 50, 51, 53, 54,
    57, 59, 65, 110
glutamic acid, 62
glutamine, 111
glycine, 51, 53, 54, 57
grants, 123
gray matter, 72, 122, 125, 128, 177
grouping, 41
growth, 3, 40, 43, 49, 65, 92, 159, 175
growth factor, 40, 43, 49, 65, 159, 175
guidelines, 123, 124

H

Hawaii, 29
headache, 5, 14, 111, 124, 125, 138, 140,
    141
healing, 41, 108, 109
health, 2, 86, 103, 106, 109, 121, 124, 186,
    189, 192, 193
health care, 2
heat loss, 17
heat stroke, 17
helplessness, 70
hemisphere, 81
hemoglobin, 71
herpes, 62, 109, 124
herpes simplex, 62
herpes zoster, 109, 124
hippocampus, 38, 39, 119
histamine, 36
histology, 175
histone, 44
histone deacetylase, 44
history, 71, 124, 136, 141, 142, 178, 188
homeostasis, 59, 108
Hong Kong, 191
house, 190

human, xiii, xv, xvi, xix, xx, 3, 13, 16, 18,
    19, 22, 25, 26, 44, 65, 67, 74, 75, 79, 84,
    86, 87, 90, 104, 105, 110, 113, 117, 124,
    125, 126, 127, 128, 129, 150, 160, 168,
    173, 176, 179, 180, 186, 189, 192, 193
human brain, xiii, xix, xx, 74, 84, 86, 110,
    117, 125, 128, 179
human cerebral cortex, 75
human development, 186, 189, 192, 193
human immunodeficiency virus, (HIV), 10,
    15, 29, 44
human subjects, 19, 86
humanistic perspective, 193
Hungary, 3
Hunter, 81, 88
hydrolysis, 9
hyperactivity, 56
hypersensitivity, 11, 16, 44, 45, 46, 63, 65,
    173
hyperthermia, 2, 17, 18, 23, 30, 32
hypertrophy, 159
hypnosis, 72, 73
hypothalamus, 73, 137, 150
hypothermia, 18
hypothesis, 9, 26, 124, 158, 163
hypothyroidism, 154, 172

I

IASP, 74, 108, 123, 128
identification, 16, 22, 41
idiopathic, 86, 108, 123, 159, 174, 175, 178
illusion, 83, 100, 103, 106
image, 46, 80, 82, 87, 110
imagery, xx, 77, 81, 82, 85, 89, 92, 95, 96,
    97, 98, 99, 100, 102, 103, 104, 105, 106
images, 71, 95, 103, 124
imagination, 95, 106
imaging modalities, 158
immersion, 19
immobilization, 171
immune system, 59
immunoreactivity, 65
implants, 146, 148
improvements, 80, 142, 164, 166

Index

impulses, 161
in vitro, 11, 16, 27, 28, 31
in vivo, 10, 11, 16, 24, 27, 30, 31, 45, 65, 67, 104, 110, 127
incidence, 94, 108, 109, 123, 124, 174
India, 3
individuals, 19, 21, 90, 125
induction, 6, 39, 44, 75, 133, 170
industry, 22
infarction, 133, 142
infection, 109, 138, 141
inflammation, 1, 3, 5, 6, 7, 20, 23, 25, 30, 45, 60, 66, 70, 159, 179
inflammatory bowel disease, 7
inflammatory cells, 159
inflammatory mediators, 9, 58
inguinal, 14
inguinal hernia, 14
inhibition, xvi, 12, 38, 40, 41, 52, 57, 60, 62, 63, 73, 90, 114, 127, 150
inhibitor, 16, 61
initiation, 21, 164
injections, 2, 10, 13, 22, 178
injury, xvi, 1, 5, 11, 13, 19, 20, 21, 23, 29, 30, 34, 35, 36, 40, 41, 42, 43, 44, 45, 46, 57, 59, 61, 65, 66, 67, 70, 78, 86, 92, 94, 103, 106, 109, 135, 142, 149, 155, 156, 157, 173, 174, 178
inositol, 65
insertion, 38
integration, 48, 72, 110, 119, 128, 165
intellectual disabilities, 193
interference, 4, 11, 24
international meetings, 185
interneurons, 48, 50, 51, 52, 56, 64
intervention, 1, 2, 28, 81, 97, 99, 102
intestine, 11
intravenously, 18
investors, 24, 25, 32
ion channels, 7, 26, 38, 53, 64
ions, 53
ipsilateral, 82, 98, 102, 114, 115, 119, 121
ischemia, 5, 20, 156, 157, 179
isolation, 103
isotope, 110

Israel, xii, xv, xix, 33, 131, 185, 186, 187, 188, 189, 190, 192, 193
issues, xvi, 22, 193
Italy, 1

J

Japan, 5, 21
joint pain, 16, 31

K

kinase activity, 55
kinetics, 30
Kinsey, 26
knee arthroplasty, 13

L

laminar, 113
latency, 158, 159, 162, 166, 167
lateral epicondylitis, 14, 29
laterality, 82, 100
lead, xiii, xx, 4, 16, 34, 70, 78, 92, 136, 140, 141, 142, 146, 147, 162, 163
learning, 73, 79, 112, 160, 165, 169, 175
lesions, 72, 76, 109, 165
ligand, 53
light, 10, 34, 47, 49, 59, 71, 102, 108, 113, 114, 116, 118, 120
limbic system, 111, 179
linoleic acid, 7, 26
local anesthesia, 3
local anesthetic, 61
locus, 52, 73
longitudinal study, 172
lower limb amputees, 81

M

magnesium, 39
magnetic resonance, 71, 74, 76, 82, 86, 105, 125, 126, 127, 151, 155, 179, 180

Index

magnetic resonance imaging (MRI), 71, 74, 75, 76, 82, 86, 105, 111, 126, 133, 151, 154, 155, 158, 159, 168, 179, 180
magnetic resonance spectroscopy, 125, 127
magnetoencephalography, 110, 154, 161
magnitude, 15
major depressive disorder, 73, 74
majority, 15
man, 11, 17, 76, 86, 104, 126, 149, 175
management, 13, 14, 91, 95, 99, 103, 123, 124, 132, 136, 150, 169, 173, 178
manipulation, 79, 95, 169, 170
mapping, 105, 126, 128
Marani, 177
mass, 162, 168
matrix, 102, 125
matter, 117, 125, 126
MCP, 44
MCP-1, 44
measurement, 82, 110
measurements, 166
mechanical stress, 156
media, 25
median, 84, 153, 154, 155, 156, 157, 158, 159, 160, 161, 162, 163, 164, 165, 166, 167, 168, 169, 171, 173, 174, 175, 177, 178
mediation, 23, 39
medical, 47, 70, 110, 132, 148, 185, 186, 188
medication, 61, 62, 140, 147, 148
medicine, xvi, xvii, 3, 90, 192
medulla, 72
MEG, 71, 98, 110, 121, 122, 154, 161, 164, 175
membranes, 53
memory, 44, 54, 95, 97, 106, 117, 118, 119, 169, 180
memory formation, 118, 180
meningioma, 143
mental health, 165
mental image, xi, 89, 91, 95, 96, 99, 100, 102, 103, 104, 105, 106
mental representation, 96, 104
messengers, 54

meta-analysis, 71, 72, 76, 166
metabolic pathways, 110
metabolism, 40, 110
metabolites, 7, 26, 110
metatarsal, 170
methodology, 125
Mexico, 32
mice, 11, 17, 19, 24, 28, 31, 44, 64
middle frontal gyrus, 117
migraine headache, 14, 29
mission, 187, 189
mitogen, 38, 40, 46, 54
models, 4, 9, 16, 17, 22, 30, 41, 45, 55, 57, 59, 60, 61, 62, 67, 109, 110, 124, 156, 157, 159, 160, 161, 169
modern science, 3
modifications, xx, 48
molecular biology, 150
molecules, 6, 11, 12, 13, 26, 53, 60, 110
Montana, 65
mood disorder, 70, 76, 117
Moon, 28
morbidity, 140, 170
morphine, 27, 46, 66
morphology, 115
motivation, 70, 72
motor activity, 97
motor control, 88, 104, 164, 165
Motor Cortex Stimulation (MCS), 133, 138
motor skills, 95
motor system, 87, 97, 104, 105
motor task, 94, 96, 97
mRNA, 28, 64
multidimensional, 128
multiple factors, 165
multiple sclerosis, 133, 135, 136, 140, 150
multipotent, 60
muscle relaxant, 135
muscle strain, 13
muscles, 96, 104, 164
musicians, 94, 104
myelin, 159
myositis, 44

N

N-acetyl-aspartate (NAA), 110
National Institutes of Health, 63, 186
Native Americans, 3
nausea, 143
NCS, 155, 158, 166
necrosis, 26, 41, 45
neonates, 44
nerve, 3, 8, 10, 11, 13, 23, 28, 29, 34, 40, 41, 42, 43, 45, 46, 48, 49, 51, 55, 57, 59, 60, 65, 66, 67, 80, 90, 97, 124, 134, 135, 140, 142, 153, 154, 155, 156, 157, 158, 159, 160, 161, 162, 163, 164, 165, 166, 167, 168, 169, 171, 172, 173, 174, 175, 178, 179
nerve conduction velocity, 174
nerve fibers, 3, 28, 41, 49
nerve growth factor, 8, 49, 65, 66
nervous system, xvi, 48, 52, 59, 63, 86, 92, 93, 94, 126
neural connection, 93
neural network, xiii, xx, 70, 92, 169
neuralgia, 3, 5, 13, 14, 21, 29, 66, 109, 123, 124, 135, 141, 142, 146
neurocognitive testing, xx
neurodegenerative disorders, 117
neuroendocrine cells, 41
neuroimaging, xi, xiii, xvi, xix, xx, 69, 70, 71, 73, 75, 76, 103, 107, 110, 111, 122, 154, 156, 163, 179
neuroinflammation, 45
neurokinin, 7, 37, 64
neurological disease, 169, 171
neurological rehabilitation, 169
neuroma, 14, 28
neuronal circuits, 170
neuronal systems, 112
neurons, xv, 1, 6, 7, 9, 10, 17, 21, 22, 23, 25, 27, 28, 30, 31, 38, 39, 40, 41, 43, 44, 45, 48, 49, 50, 51, 52, 53, 54, 55, 56, 57, 58, 59, 64, 66, 67, 74, 104, 133, 134, 160, 161, 169, 176
neuropathic pain, xii, 2, 10, 11, 12, 13, 14, 16, 20, 21, 22, 29, 30, 34, 35, 36, 40, 41, 44, 45, 46, 47, 49, 62, 65, 66, 95, 102, 103, 104, 106, 107, 108, 109, 111, 112, 114, 119, 120, 121, 122, 123, 126, 128, 129, 132, 135, 136, 140, 141, 142, 143, 144, 146, 147, 148, 149, 150, 151, 152, 159, 165, 170, 173
neuropathy, 17, 29, 45, 136, 144, 153, 154, 177
neuropeptides, 7, 10, 49, 51, 55, 56, 58, 60
neurophysiology, 151
neuroscience, xvi, 104, 186
neurotoxicity, 10
neurotransmission, 53, 54, 65, 111
neurotransmitter, 36, 40, 49, 52, 54, 92
neurotransmitters, 47, 49, 51, 54, 56, 58, 60
neurotrophic factors, 55, 59
neutral, 166
next generation, 23, 192
nicotine, 3
nitric oxide, 57, 58, 59
nitric oxide synthase, 57
NMDA receptors, 37, 38, 57, 176
Nobel Prize, 186
nonconscious, 76
non-oncologic patient populations, 4
norepinephrine, 12, 51, 52, 62
Norway, 191
NSAIDs, 166
nuclei, 72, 110, 115
nucleus, 18, 52, 73, 110, 117, 136, 137, 140, 175
null, 11

O

obesity, 154, 171
oculomotor, 105
oil, 8
oligodendrocytes, 40
opioids, 51, 52, 62, 66, 76, 135
opportunities, xx, 1
optimism, 22
optimization, 4
organism, 48, 108
oscillatory activity, 170

204 Index

osteoarthritis, 5, 13, 14, 28, 154
overlap, 79

P

Pacific, 191
paclitaxel, 61, 67
pain management, xx, 13, 16, 31, 99, 132,
 135, 146, 185
pairing, 80, 86, 176
parallel, xv, 28, 40, 70
parenchyma, 45
paresthesias, 34, 155, 156, 157, 158, 161,
 162, 163, 164, 167, 173
parietal cortex, 112, 119, 149
parietal lobe, 98
participants, 21, 100, 102, 146
patents, 2
pathogenesis, 7
pathology, xv, 70
pathophysiological, 30, 155, 157
pathophysiology, xx, 104, 108, 109, 154,
 156, 158
pathways, xvi, 4, 37, 38, 39, 44, 48, 50, 51,
 52, 54, 62, 64, 70, 71, 72, 73, 93, 96, 99,
 102, 157, 175, 180
peer review, 185, 186
peptide, 7, 10, 37, 49, 167, 179
peptides, 44, 167
perceptual learning, 87, 88
perceptual performance, 171
peripheral nervous system, 43, 70, 91
peripheral neuropathy, 171
permeability, 53
permit, 39
PET scan, 71
PGE, 159
phantom limb pain, 78, 79, 80, 81, 82, 83,
 87, 88, 89, 90, 95, 100, 106, 149
pharmaceutical, 4, 16, 22
pharmaceuticals, 25, 32
pharmacological treatment, 135, 148
pharmacology, 3, 32, 64, 65
pharmacotherapy, 92
phenomenology, xx, 104

phenotype, 11, 60
phenotypes, 11, 28
Philadelphia, 1, 123
phosphate, 65
phosphoinositides, 27
phosphorylation, 9, 26, 27, 39, 52, 56, 58,
 65
photographs, 100
physical interaction, 49
physicians, 6
physiological, 64
physiological mechanisms, 185
physiology, xv, xx, 49
pilot study, 29, 89, 101, 149, 151
placebo, 14, 20, 21, 22, 28, 29, 63, 66, 71,
 72, 73, 76, 110, 150, 152, 179
plaque, 135
plasma membrane, 27
plasticity, xi, xiii, xix, 10, 33, 39, 43, 44, 47,
 48, 49, 55, 56, 59, 63, 70, 73, 78, 85, 86,
 87, 91, 92, 93, 94, 99, 103, 104, 106,
 113, 126, 160, 161, 163, 167, 169, 170,
 173, 175, 176
Plato, 95
plexus, 143
PLP, 95, 100
policy, 192
polypeptide, 59
population, 2, 40, 47, 59, 70, 83, 102, 108,
 123, 136, 143, 147, 172, 174
positive feedback, 156
positron, 71, 74, 76, 116, 127, 129
positron emission tomography (PET), 71,
 74, 75, 76, 110, 116, 121, 122, 127, 128,
 129
potassium, 41, 44, 53
prefrontal cortex, 73, 82, 115, 116, 119,
 122, 127
pregnancy, 154
preparation, 13, 97
pressure pain threshold (PPT), 163
prevention, 23, 186
primate, 104, 180
principles, 86
probability, 8

Index

professionals, 190, 192
prognosis, 107
pro-inflammatory, 7, 8, 10, 41, 67
project, 85, 192
proliferation, 159, 160, 175
propagation, 42, 48
prostaglandins, 8, 9, 36, 58
prostheses, 78, 85
prosthesis, 80, 84, 87
prosthetic device, 80
protective role, 46, 65
protein kinase C, 9, 26, 38, 54, 57, 66
protein kinases, 54, 55, 57, 173
protein synthesis, 38, 70
proteins, 39
protons, 8, 16, 20, 26, 36, 110
psychology, 95, 185
public health, 189, 190, 192
public service, 189
pumps, 12
punishment, 115

Q

quality of life, 124, 140, 186, 193
quantitative sensory testing, xx

R

radius, 154
rash, 109
reactions, 57
reactivity, 73
reality, xx, 83, 85, 89, 90
recall, 95
recall information, 95
receptive field, 80, 126, 168, 170
receptors, 8, 10, 12, 16, 25, 26, 28, 31, 38,
    40, 44, 45, 48, 49, 50, 51, 52, 53, 54, 55,
    57, 58, 59, 60, 61, 62, 64, 65, 66, 73, 76,
    103, 125, 158, 160, 161, 174
recognition, 82, 93, 100, 112, 170
reconstruction, 111
recovery, 65, 86, 87, 95, 99, 149, 178

redistribution, 78
regression, 41
rehabilitation, 85, 89, 90, 99, 149, 186, 189
reinforcers, 115
relaxation, 75, 83
relief, xi, 1, 2, 4, 10, 13, 14, 15, 21, 22, 23,
    24, 27, 29, 66, 76, 84, 95, 101, 102, 103,
    107, 115, 122, 132, 133, 136, 140, 141,
    142, 144, 146, 148, 151, 152, 156, 166
religion, 100
remyelination, 175
repair, 14, 59, 102, 165
requirements, 7
research funding, 85
researchers, xv, 47, 63, 71, 72, 92, 98, 193
resistance, 91, 112
resolution, 110, 121, 122, 139, 142, 172,
    174
respiratory arrest, 22
respiratory rate, 96
response, xiii, xv, xx, 7, 11, 12, 15, 17, 18,
    19, 20, 22, 34, 35, 36, 37, 38, 40, 43, 49,
    53, 57, 66, 70, 71, 72, 73, 74, 91, 92, 93,
    98, 99, 100, 102, 106, 110, 118, 121,
    144, 155, 156, 160, 161, 165, 168, 171,
    180
responsiveness, 27
restitution, 78
restoration, 151
reticulum, 39
retina, 158
rheumatoid arthritis, 13, 159
risk, 2, 21, 23, 127, 148, 154, 170, 172
risk factors, 172
risks, 140
RNA, 4, 6, 11, 24
RNAi, 6, 24
rodents, 19, 26, 28
root, 7, 41, 43, 45, 49, 65, 67, 109, 124, 135,
    142, 179
roots, 3, 100
rubber, 83, 90
rules, 96

S

sadness, 111
safety, 2, 14, 21, 66
scavengers, 59
school, 192
science, xv, xvi, xvii, 63, 88, 104, 169, 171, 179, 190
scientific papers, 3
scope, 156
secrete, 49, 59
secretion, 49, 55, 60
seizure, 138, 139, 180
selectivity, 6, 16, 25, 65
self-regulation, 72, 73
sensation, 2, 7, 15, 19, 24, 25, 28, 34, 35, 73, 75, 81, 82, 83, 88, 96, 100, 101, 111, 122, 128, 129, 140, 143, 157, 170
sensations, 34, 78, 83, 84, 96, 97, 100, 121, 134, 153, 161
senses, 81
sensitivity, 7, 11, 20, 27, 30, 43, 54, 78, 86, 110, 158, 177
sensitization, 9, 26, 34, 35, 36, 37, 38, 39, 40, 41, 43, 44, 48, 49, 63, 66, 67, 155, 159, 173, 177
sensors, 17, 29
sensory experience, 70
sensory modalities, 93
sensory symptoms, 155, 177
serine, 53
serotonin, 12, 36, 51, 52, 62
serum, 174
sex, 124
sham stimulation, 139, 166
shape, 160
shingles, 124, 135
showing, 101, 144, 159
side effects, 12, 41, 60, 61, 62, 135, 137, 140
signal transduction, 65
signaling pathway, 26, 39, 59
signalling, 11
signals, 34, 39, 40, 47, 48, 49, 50, 51, 52, 53, 55, 59, 70, 92, 97, 105, 120

signs, 33, 34, 36, 109, 158, 159
Sinai, 33, 69
skeletal muscle, 179
skin, 7, 10, 13, 17, 19, 34, 36, 80, 108, 121, 122, 124, 126, 160, 179
smooth muscle, 25
society, 63, 190
sodium, 22, 38, 41, 42, 43, 53, 61, 159, 175
solution, 21
somata, 7
somatosensory cortex, 7, 75, 79, 80, 86, 87, 104, 105, 112, 113, 114, 121, 122, 126, 132, 135, 148, 154, 162, 168, 176, 177, 179
specialists, 188
species, 11, 16, 17, 19
spectroscopy, 125
speech, 139, 141, 142
spiders, 8
spinal cord, 16, 18, 26, 35, 39, 41, 44, 45, 46, 47, 48, 62, 64, 67, 70, 72, 92, 94, 100, 102, 103, 105, 106, 127, 133, 144, 149, 156, 173
spinal cord injury, 46, 94, 100, 102, 105, 106, 127, 133, 149
spine, 104
splinting, 156, 165, 166, 173, 178
Spring, 17
sprouting, 49, 55, 56, 60, 65, 70, 114
standard deviation, 158
state, 2, 7, 9, 22, 53, 70, 88, 92, 96, 100, 106, 161
states, 3, 7, 11, 16, 37, 41, 49, 55, 66, 73, 77, 78, 96, 128, 160, 161, 169
steroids, 135, 156, 165, 166
stimulus, xvi, 9, 16, 22, 34, 43, 49, 108, 110, 121, 128
stress, 67, 70, 110, 117, 175
stroke, 77, 81, 86, 88, 95, 96, 99, 105, 106, 135, 141, 142, 144, 146
structural changes, 78, 111, 112, 122, 158
structure, 7, 15, 71, 117, 156
suppression, 166
surgical intervention, 154
survival, 48

Index

survivors, 43
Sweden, 191
swelling, 139, 158, 159, 160
Switzerland, 24
symptoms, xvi, 4, 33, 34, 84, 103, 109, 134, 143, 155, 156, 164, 165, 166, 172, 173
synapse, 39, 47, 50, 55, 65, 103, 175
synaptic clefts, 50
synaptic plasticity, 35, 38, 64, 161, 169, 180
synaptic strength, 162
synaptic transmission, 46, 53, 64
synchronization, 169, 170
syndrome, 78, 79, 84, 87, 89, 95, 100, 133, 141, 146, 148, 149, 153, 154, 160, 172, 174, 175, 177, 179, 193
synthesis, 39
systemic lupus erythematosus, 159

T

tactile stimuli, 80
target, 4, 5, 6, 9, 12, 17, 27, 32, 77, 122, 135, 144, 169
task performance, 165
techniques, 71, 90, 95, 110, 121, 132, 133, 134, 135, 143, 144, 147, 154, 170, 171, 187
technologies, 132
technology, 89
teeth, 3
temperature, 4, 17, 18, 19, 21, 22, 25, 29, 31, 34, 36
temporal lobe, 119, 128
temporal lobe epilepsy, 128
tenosynovitis, 155
tension, 111, 125
terminals, 35, 47, 50, 51, 52, 55, 57, 59, 65
territory, 140, 160, 163
testing, xx, 22, 140, 142, 157, 158, 163, 165
textbook, 123
TGF, 159
thalamus, 37, 48, 71, 74, 102, 111, 132, 133, 135, 140
therapeutic approaches, 4, 23, 75, 164
therapeutic effects, 106

therapeutic interventions, 154
therapeutic use, 26, 99
therapeutics, 32, 67
therapy, 10, 23, 24, 66, 76, 82, 88, 95, 99, 100, 101, 103, 106, 147, 150, 165, 166, 167, 173
thermoregulation, 18, 31
thermosensation, 1, 27
thinning, 111, 114, 115, 117, 118, 119, 120
third molar, 20, 21
thyroid, 172
tin, 155
tinnitus, 77
tissue, 1, 5, 10, 12, 20, 30, 35, 41, 48, 59, 71, 108, 120, 160, 175
TLR, 58, 59
TLR4, 40, 62
TNF, 8, 41, 56, 59, 60, 61, 159
TNF-alpha, 8
TNF-α, 56, 159
tonic, 128
tooth, 3, 20, 114, 120, 126
topical anesthetic, 170
toxicity, 15
toxin, 25
trafficking, 27, 57
training, xi, xx, 77, 78, 80, 81, 82, 83, 84, 87, 100, 102, 105, 106, 126, 161, 185, 186
transcription, 38
transducer, 1
transduction, 1
transection, 165
transformation, 55
translocation, 58
transmission, xvi, 38, 42, 43, 44, 48, 50, 52, 54, 56, 67, 73
transplant, 65
trauma, 94, 109, 135, 141, 143, 170
treatment, xii, xx, 2, 10, 14, 15, 16, 20, 21, 22, 24, 29, 31, 44, 49, 60, 61, 62, 63, 66, 67, 73, 76, 78, 82, 85, 89, 90, 100, 103, 108, 112, 122, 123, 125, 127, 131, 132, 133, 134, 135, 136, 140, 142, 144, 145, 146, 147, 148, 149, 150, 151, 152, 154,

155, 164, 165, 166, 167, 168, 169, 170, 171, 173, 179, 185, 193
trial, 5, 13, 14, 15, 16, 20, 21, 28, 29, 61, 62, 67, 81, 88, 89, 100, 106, 127, 128, 139, 142, 149, 166, 173, 178, 181
trigeminal nerve, 109, 134, 135, 136, 140, 141, 142, 143, 144, 147
trigeminal neuralgia, 12, 84, 108, 112, 114, 116, 120, 123, 124, 125, 126, 135, 136, 141, 142, 146, 147, 148, 150, 152
TRPV1 antagonists, 2, 3, 4, 10, 15, 16, 17, 18, 19, 20, 21, 22, 23, 24, 31, 32
tumor, 8, 41, 46, 56, 58, 109
tumor necrosis factor, 8, 41, 46, 56, 58
type 2 diabetes, 65
tyrosine, 39, 55

validation, 4
vanilloid (capsaicin) receptor, 1, 7, 21
variables, 144
vasodilation, 17, 179
vector, 62
velocity, 122, 166, 174
vibration, 155, 170
virology, 124
virtual reality (VR), 83
viscera, 32
vision, 81, 93, 97
visual area, 112
visual system, 97
visualization, 81
voiding, 6
vomiting, 143

U

ultrasonography, 172
ultrasound, 155, 156, 158, 159, 165
unique features, 122
united, xix, 1, 2, 33, 47, 69, 91, 107, 124, 131, 186, 188, 191
United Kingdom (UK), 91, 123, 191
United States, xix, 1, 2, 33, 47, 69, 107, 124, 131, 186, 188
urea, 16, 30, 31
urinary tract, 27
USA, 26, 27, 32, 75, 105, 153

W

walking, 103
Washington, 30
water, 19, 21, 158
water diffusion, 158
weakness, 155, 156, 164
weapons, 3
welfare, 186, 189
well-being, 186
white matter, 72
withdrawal, 2, 11, 19
workers, 155, 172
working memory, 76
worldwide, 140
wound infection, 138, 139, 142

V

vagus, 26
vagus nerve, 26